AVIAN PATHOLOGY

About the Authors

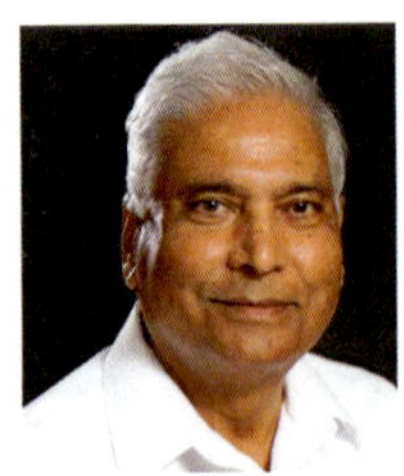

Dr. Ravindra Nath Sharma born at Allahabad, Uttar Pradesh, a veterinary graduate of 1961 class from the U.P. College of Veterinary Medicine Mathura, obtained MSc and PhD in Veterinary Pathology from the Indian Veterinary Research Institute (IVRI), Izatnagar in 1965 and 1974 respectively.

Dr. Sharma is recipient of the "Jawahar Lal Nehru" award for 1975 for the development of diagnostic reagents for Marek's disease suitable for India. Recently, in 2008 he was awarded Pfizer research excellence award for his research contribution. In 2016, he was honored as fellow of the Indian Association of Veterinary pathologists. In 1976, selection of Dr. Sharma, from candidates of 39 Commonwealth countries, as consultant (poultry Pathologist) to the Commonwealth fund for technical cooperation (CFTC) was viewed as great honor for the IVRI and the country as a whole. During 4 year mission of CFTC in Zambia, his research findings made Zambia free of major poultry diseases.

Because of his vast experience and vision in Veterinary Pathology, he served in five prestigious universities, three in Asian continent (India, Iran and Libya), one in Africa (Zambia) and currently working with one in West Indies. Through out his carrier in these universities, he taught and conducted research in Pathology and avian diseases.

Currently, Dr. Sharma is serving as professor of pathology and avian diseases, Associate Dean School of Graduate Studies and Associate Director Research at the school of veterinary medicine, St. George's University, Grenada.

Dr. Sharma has mentored more than 2 dozen students for their PhD and MSc degree in Veterinary Pathology and avian diseases. He has written a book, 3 monographs and published more than 200 research papers. He has made more than 20 presentations at international scientific meetings.

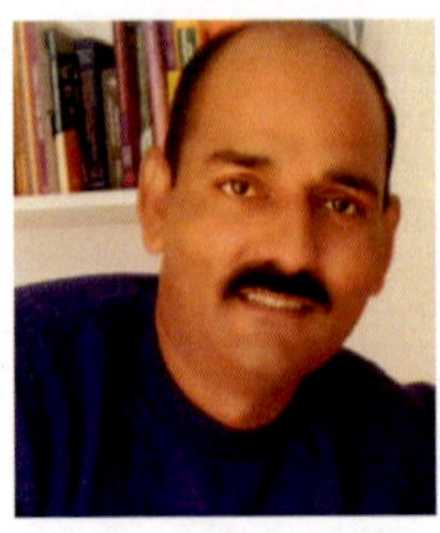

Dr. Neelesh Sharma is graduated in Veterinary Science in 2001 and post-graduated in Veterinary Medicine in 2003. Dr Sharma focused on Stem cell based research in livestock during Ph.D. from Jeju National University, South Korea; and presently working as Senior Assistant Professor in the Division of Veterinary Medicine, Faculty of Veterinary Science & Animal Husbandry, Sher-e-Kashmir University of Agricultural Sciences & Technology of Jammu (SKUAST-J), India. He has more than 13 years experience in teaching, research and extension. Dr. Sharma is actively involved in the teaching of Veterinary undergraduate, post-graduate and PhD students. He is also working on different research projects.

Dr. Sharma is a "*ICAR-International Fellow*". He has travelled to many countries and delivered invited lectures in the international conferences, symposia, seminars etc. He has bestowed with numerous National and International awards such as The Bronze Standard International Award by HRH The Duke of Edinburgh, UK; NAAS Associateship, Graduate student award, Beijing China; Outstanding Presentation Award, South Korea; Outstanding Research Scholarship award, Thailand; Dr. D.C. Blood Gold Medal Award, IAAVR Merit Award etc. and recipient of various best poster/presentation awards at national and international level. Dr. Sharma has authored/edited 10 books/compendiums and >140 papers in journals of repute. Dr. Sharma is founder Editor-In-Chief, Journal of Animal Research having NAAS rating 5.68 (2017) and technical editor/regional editor/editorial board member of about 20 scientific journals. He is member of various scientific societies and has attended many conferences at National and International level.

AVIAN PATHOLOGY

Dr. Ravindra Nath Sharma
Professor of Pathology and Avian Diseases
School of Veterinary Medicine
St. George's University
Grenada, West Indies

Dr. Neelesh Sharma
Senior Assistant Professor
Division of Veterinary Medicine
F.V.Sc. & A.H., SKUAST-Jammu
R.S. Pura, Jammu, India

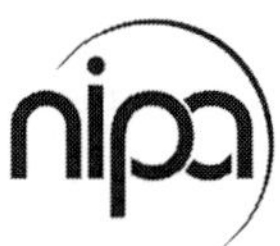

NEW INDIA PUBLISHING AGENCY
New Delhi – 110 034

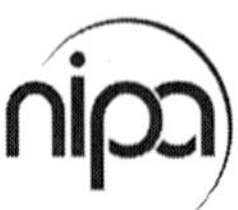

NEW INDIA PUBLISHING AGENCY
101, Vikas Surya Plaza, CU Block, LSC Market
Pitam Pura, New Delhi 110 034, India
Phone: + 91 (11) 27 34 17 17 Fax: + 91 (11) 27 34 16 16
Email: info@nipabooks.com
Web: www.nipabooks.com

Feedback at feedbacks@nipabooks.com

ISBN: 978-93-87973-16-9

Composed and Designed by NIPA

DEDICATION

I would like to dedicate this book to my wife Mrs. Malti Sharma without their continued support and belief in me, this book and my work would not be possible.

Dr. Ravindra Nath Sharma

Preface

Since past few decades because of changing demand for white meat from red meat, the small poultry farms and backyard poultry units developed to commercial farms. The adaptation of intensive poultry keeping methods and rearing of different species of poultry together has given rise to many disease problems. Since the inception of intensive poultry production worldwide farmers were struggling with severe diseases and huge economic losses in their unit. In order to keep pace with ever expanding poultry industry and meeting the increased demand for poultry products, knowledge for prevention and control of poultry diseases will be crucial.

Realizing the importance of the knowledge of poultry diseases for future veterinarians, Veterinary Council of India (VCI) included "Avian Pathology" course in the syllabus of graduates in Veterinary Science. Since the book is in accordance with the VCI syllabus, the book will enable veterinary students to have sound understanding and working knowledge of poultry diseases. I hope the students will find this book a useful learning. The book will also assist personnel at the poultry disease diagnostic laboratories and progressive farmers.

The book devotes total seven sections including basics about avian, bacterial diseases, viral diseases, fungal diseases, parasitic diseases, nutritional deficiency diseases and miscellaneous disorders affecting poultry. There are total 55 chapters in a capsule form. Emphasis has been put on etiology, transmission, epizootiology, clinical signs, gross and microscopic lesions, diagnosis, treatment and control. Where necessary, mention has been made on zoonoses. Necessary images and tables have been added to enhance the understanding of the diseases.

I thankfully acknowledge the source of images taken from American Association of Avian Pathologists continuing education program- slide study sets, a color atlas of diseases of domestic fowl and turkey; by C.J. Randall 1st edn. (1987) Wolfe medical publication ltd, Self assessment color review of avian medicine by R.B. Altman and N. A. Forbes, Iowa state university press and contribution by students of veterinary medicine at St George's University Grenada.

I appreciate the help of Dr. Keshaw P. Tiwari, Assistant Professor, Department of Veterinary Pathology, School of Veterinary Medicine, St George's University, Grenada in preparation and review of the book.

Dr. Ravindra Nath Sharma
Dr. Neelesh Sharma

Contents

Section-3: Viral Diseases

Section-4: Fungal Diseases

Section-5: Parasitic Diseases

Section-6: Deficiency Diseases

Section-7: Miscellaneous Disorders

1

Glossary of Poultry Terms

A

Abdomen: Area between the keel and the pubic (hip) bones.

Abdominal capacity: The distance between the two public bones (width) and between the pubic bones and the tip of the keel (depth).

Addled: An egg where the contents are decomposing.

Air cell: The air space between the two shell membranes, usually at the large end of the egg.

Albumen: The white of an egg.

Alektorophobia: The fear of chickens.

Allantois: A sac connected to the embryo's abdomen and involved in embryo respiration.

Amnion: A sac surrounding the embry filled with amniotic fluid which protects the developing embryo from shock and provides a medium for the develop embryo to exercise their muscles.

Antibody: A natural substance in the blood that recognizes and destroys foreign invaders and that causes an immune response to vaccination or infection.

Anticoccidial: An anticoccidial drug used to treat or prevent coccidiosis.

Antigen: A foreign protein in the blood that differs from nautral body proteins and, as a result, stimulates the natural production of antibodies.

Artificial insemination: The introduction of semen into the female oviduct by methods other than by natural mating.

As hatched: Description of a group of chicks that have not been sorted.

Ascites: Accumulation of fluid in the abdominal cavity.

Aves: A class of animals composed of birds.

Avian: Pertaining to birds.

Aviary system: A 'litter system' of housing where a number of "mezzanine" floors are installed to increase the available floor space and, in doing so, provide the space for more birds in the poultry house.

Aviary: A large enclosure for holding birds in confinement.

Aviculture: The science of birds.

Axial feather: The short wing feather located between the primary and secondary flight feathers.

B

Banding: Putting a tag or band with identification on it to the wing or leg of a bird.

Bantam: A chicken breed that is one third to one half the size of a standard breed.

Banti: A non-technical term sometimes used to mean 'bantam'.

Barbicels: Tiny hooks that hold a feather's web together.

Barring: Alternate markings of two distinct colors on a feather.

Bay: Light golden brown in color.

Beak trimming: The removal of the tip of the beak of poultry by specially designed equipment to prevent cannibalism and its associated vices.

Beak: The hard protruding mouth part of a bird consisting of an uper and a lower part.

Beard: The feathers bunched together under the beak of some breeds of chickens; coarse hairs protruding from the breast of turkeys.

Bedding: Material scattered on the floor of a poultry house to absorb moisture and manure (also called litter).

Biddy: A non-technical term for a laying hen that is over one year of age

Bill: The 'beak' of waterfowl.

Billing out: The act of chickens using their beaks to scoop feed out of a feeder and onto the floor.

Biosecurity: Disease prevention program.

Bird: The term often used to refer to an individual of any breed of poultry.

Blade: The lower, smooth part of a single comb.

Blastoderm: The fertilised nucleus of the egg from which the chicken develops.

Blastodisc: The unfertilised nucleus of an egg. No chicken can develop from a blastodisc.

Bleaching: The disappearance of the color from the vent, face and shanks of yellow-skinned chickens.

Blood spot: Blood in an egg.

Bloom: The moist protective coating on a freshly laid eggs that partially seals the pores of the egg shell to prevent penetration by bacteria (also called the cuticle).

Blowout: When there is vent damage, typically caused by laying a very large egg (also referred to as a prolapse).

Blue: Slate gray feather color.

Booted: Having feathers on the shanks (legs) and toes.

Bow-legged: Deformity in which legs are farther apart at hocks than at feet.

Breast blister: enlarged, discolored area on the breast or keel bone often seen in heavy birds.

Breed: A group of birds that reproduce their own likeness in their offspring. A variety is a group within a breed that are distinguished by a difference of a single characteristic eg. feather colour or comb type.

Broiler: A young bird of either sex that is bred and grown specifically for highly efficient meat production. Broilers are usually grown for 5 to 7 weeks of age (alternative term – meat chicken).

Brood: A group of chicks of same age raised in one batch is called as a brood.

Brooder: The equipment used to provide supplementary warmth during the early stages of the chickens' life. The energy used may come from electricity, gas, oil or from other sources.

Brooding: The period of the first weeks of a chicken's life when it requires a very high standard of care including the provision of special diets and supplementary warmth.

Broody: The instinct controlled by maternal hormones that causes the female to want to sit on eggs for hatching and to care for the chickens that hatch.

Buff: Orange-yellow color in feathers that is not shiny or brassy.

C

Caeca: The two blind gut of the digestive tract attached to the distal end of the small intestine.

Cages: A system of housing where the birds are confined to a wire floor singly or in multiples. With this system the stock do not come into contact with their own or other bird's faeces which is an important disease control measure.

Candle: To assess some internal characteristics of the egg by viewing it in a darkened room with a bright light behind the egg.

Candler: Light used to examine the contents of an egg without breaking it open.

Candling: Using a candler to check the contents of an egg.

Cannibalism: The practice by some birds of attacking and eating other members of the same flock.

Cape: Narrow feathers between a chicken's neck and back.

Capon: A castrated male chicken (requires surgery since the reproductive organs are internal.

Capon: It is a young male birds of which testicle are removed.

Carrier: An apparently healthy bird that can transmit a disease to others; also refers to a container to transport birds.

Caruncle: Brigh tly colored growths on the throat region of turkeys and the face of muscovy ducks.

Chalza: Two white cords of tightly spun albumen (egg white) found on either side of the yolk and important in keeping the yolk properly positioned within the egg (plural = chalazae).

Chick: The term used to describe chickens from day old to the end of brooding.

Chick-type drinker: A drinker that is more suitable for young chickens to access water.

Chick-type feeder: A feeder that is more suitable for young chickens to access food.

Chook: An Australian term for chicken that has been used in the US for chickens in a small flock.

Chorion: A membrane the surrounds the yolk sac and amnion.

Clean legged: Having no feathers on the shanks or toes.

Clear eggs: Infertile eggs (containing no embryos) usually removed from the incubator during incubation.

Cloaca: The common external opening for the digestive, urinary and reproductive tracts of the fowl.

Clubbed down: A condition where the down feathers do not erupt from their feather sheath resulting in a coil-like appearance.

Cluck: Sound a hen makes after laying an egg.

Clutch: A group of eggs or chicks.

Clutch: The number of eggs laid by a bird on consecutive days. A clutch of 3-4 eggs is preferred.

Coccidiostat: A drug usually added to the feed and used to prevent the disease coccidiosis.

Cock: A male that has finished one season as a breeder. Usually refers to older birds.

Cockerel: A young male from day old to the end of it's first year of breeding. Often used to refer to young males up to 6 months of age.

Controlled environment housing: An intensive housing system where the operator can control temperature, air quality and light.

Coop: The house or cage in which poultry are housed.

Coverts: Feathers that cover the primary and secondary wing feathers.

Crest: Ball of feathers on the heads of some breeds of chickens and geese.

Crop: An organ, a part of the oesophagus, located at the base of the neck and used as a storage place for food after eating but before digestion.

Crossbred: A bird with parents of two or more different genotypes (or breeds or varieties).

Crude protein: The nitrogen sources in feed. It is not true protein, as nitrogen is found in dietary compounds other than protein.

Crumbles: A poultry feed that has been pelleted and then the pellets broken up.

Cuckoo: A course and irregular barring pattern in feathers.

Culling: The identification and removal of non-productive birds from the flock.

Cuticle: The outer membrane or bloom on the egg's shell.

Cygnet: Young (baby) swan.

D

Day-old chick: Hatched out chick is called as day-old-chick up to 24 hours.

Dead-in-shell: Chicks that fail to hatch from the egg.

Deep litter: The system of housing where a suitable material called litter is provided on the poultry house floor for the birds to live on.

Defect: Any characteristic that makes a chicken less than perfect.

Depopulate: To destroy an entire flock.

Dewlap: The flap of skin below the beak of turkeys and some geese.

Disease: Any condition that affects the proper functioning of the bird's system(s), organ(s) or tissue(s).

Disinfect: Kill bacteria through chemical means.

Disqualification: A defect or deformity serious enough to bar a bird from a poultry show.

Down: A layer of feathers found under the tough exterior feathers.

Drake: An adult male duck.

Dressed: Cleaned in preparation for eating (feathers and guts removed).

Droppings: Another term for chicken manure.

Dry bulb thermometer: A thermometer with a dry, uncovered bulb used to measure temperature.

Dub: To surgically remove a bird's comb and wattles close to the head.

Duck foot: A disqualification of chickens where the hind toe is carried too far forward and touches the third toe or is carried too far back and touches the ground.

Duckling: A young (baby) duck.

Duodenal loop: The upper part of the small intestine (also referred to as the duodenum)

Dust bath: The habit of chickens to splash around in soft soil to clean their feathers and discourage external Parasites.

E

Ear lobes: the flesh patch of bare skin located below the ears of birds.

Ectoparasite: an external parasite.

Egg bound: An afflicted hen is one that is unable to complete the egg formation and laying process and retains the partially or fully formed egg in the oviduct.

Egg tooth: a tiny, hard projection on the beak of a newly hatched chick that was used by the chick to break the shell to hatch (also called a chick tooth).

Embryo: the developing cihick in an egg.

Embryology: the study of the formation and development of embryos,

Encephalitis: inflammation of the brain.

Endoparasite: an internal parasite.

Enteric: affecting the intestines.

Enteritis: inflammation of the intestines.

Esophagus: the portion of the digestive tract that moves from the mouth to the stomach.

Etiology: causes of a disease.

Evaporation: changing a liquid into vapor.

Exudate: fluid associated with an inflammation or swelling.

Exudative diathesis: accumulation of fluid (exudate) under the skin or around the heart.

F

Faking: The dishonest practice of concealing a defect or disqualification from a potential buyer or a show judge.

Feather-legged: A description of those breeds of chickens with feathers growing down their shanks.

Fecal: Pertaining to the feces.

Feces: Droppings/manure.

Feed conversion ratio: The relationship between feed production and production (eggs or growth). It is usually expressed as a ratio.

Feed hopper: A semi-automatic feeding system which has the capacity to hold food in addition to that in the feeding trough associated with the feeder.

Feral: Wild, untamed.

Fertile egg: Those eggs in which fertilisation of the blastodisc has occurred to create the blastoderm. Resulted from the joining of the female ovum and the male sperm to create the embryo.

Fertile: An egg that is fertilized and thus capable of having a chick develop (under the right environmental conditions).

Fertility: Percentage of eggs that are fertile.

Finish: The amount of fat under the skin of a meat bird.

Flight feathers: The large primary and secondary feathers of the wings.

Flighty: Excitable flock inclined to fly at the slightest provocation.

Flock: A number of birds of the same origin (genotype), age and managed in the same way.

Floor eggs: Eggs laid on the floor of the shed and not in designated nest sites/ boxes.

Fluff: Downy feathers.

Foie gras: French for 'fatty liver' and is a food product made from the liver of a duck or goose that has been specifically fattened for this purpose.

Fomite: Inanimate objects such as shipping crates, feed sacks, clothing, shoes, and tires that may harbor disease-causing organisms and thus able to transmit the disease.

Foot candle: A measurement of light intensity.

Forage: To scratch the ground in search of food; also refers to the crops in a pasture

Forced-air incubator: An incubator that has a fan to circulate warm air.

Fowl: The term used to describe all members of Gallus domesticus (domestic fowl) irrespective of age, sex or breed.

Free range housing: A system of housing where the birds have a shelter house and access to an outside area during the hours of daylight.

Frizzle: A feather that curls rather than laying flat.

Fryer: A young meat-type chicken.

G

Gander: a male goose.

Germinal disc: The fertilisation site on the egg yolk. Alternative names include blastodisc and blastoderm.

Germs: disease causing organisms.

Giblets: the parts of a chicken carcass that consist of the heart, gizzard and liver.

Gizzard: a portion of the avian digestive tract with thick muscular walls that crushes and grinds food.

Gizzard: The muscular stomach of the fowl where the food is ground and mixed with the digestive compounds produced by the proventriculus (glandular stomach).

Gobbler: an adult male turkey (also referred to as a 'tom').

Goose: a type of waterfowl; the female of the species is also referred to as a goose (the male is a gander).

Gosling: a young (baby) goose.

Grade: to sort according to quality.

Grit: small pebbles eaten by birds and used by the gizzard to grind up feed.

Growers: The term used to describe all stock between the end of brooding and till they reach sexual maturity.

Guinea cock: an adult male guinea fowl.

Guinea cockerel: a young male guinea fowl under one year of age.

Guinea hen: an adult female guinea fowl.

Guinea pullet: a female guinea fowl under one year of age.

H

Hackles: Feathers over the back of a chicken which are pointed in males and rounded in females.

Hatch of Fertile (HOF): The number of saleable chickens that hatch from all eggs classified as fertile.

Hatch: The process by which the chick comes out of the egg.

Hatchability: The number of saleable chickens that hatch from all eggs incubated – usually expressed as a percentage.

Hatchery: A place where eggs are incubated and chicks hatched.

Hen day average: Progressive egg production record calculated on a survivor basis and expressed as a percentage.

Hen feathered: The characteristic of some breeds of chickens where the male has rounded feathers (rather than pointed) like those of a female.

Hen housed average: Progressive egg production record calculated on the basis of the number of birds placed in the laying house at point of lay.

Hen: A female after the first moult. It is often used to describe females after they have started to lay.

Hock: The joint of the leg between the lower thigh and the shank. It is most commonly the region where the feathered portion of the leg ends and the scaly shank of the lower leg starts.

Horizontal transmission: Disease passed from mother to offspring via the egg.

Host: an animal that has a parasite or an infectious agent living on or in it.

Hover: A canopy used on brooders to direct the heat downwards to the chickens.

Humidity: the amount of water in the environment (usually measured with a wet bulb thermometer).

Hybrid: offspring of parents from different breeds (also referred to as crossbred); the artificial crossing of two different species.

I

Immunity: Resistance to disease (active immunity develops when an individual has had the disease or been vaccinated; passive immunity is passed from mother to chick through the egg).

Impaction: the blockage of a part of the digestive tract, typically the crop or cloaca.

Inbred: offspring of closely related parents.

Incubation period: the time it takes for an egg to hatch once incubation starts; also refers to the time from exposure to a disease causing agent to the time when the first symptoms of the disease appear.

Incubation: The process by which fertile eggs are subjected to conditions suitable for the initiation and sustaining of embryonic development and the hatching of strong, healthy chickens.

Incubator: The machine used to incubate fertile eggs.

Infectious: capable of invading living tissue and multiplying so as to cause a disease.

Infertile: an egg that is not fertilized and therefore will not hatch.

Infertility: the inability to reproduce (can be with either the male or female and can be a temporary or permanent condition).

Infundibulum: The beginning of the oviduct that picks up the ovulated yolk when it is released from the ovary (also called the funnel).

Ingest: to eat.

Insoluble grit: Hard, insoluble material such as granite, flint or bluestone chips consumed by the birds to aid in the grinding of the food in the gizzard.

Intensity of lay: how well a hen is laying right now.

Intensive system: Any system of housing poultry where the birds are indoors all of the time and do not have access to the outside. It usually entails higher stocking densities.

Intranasal: in the nose.

Intraocular: in the eye.

Intravenous: injection into a vein.

Iris: colored circle that surrounds the black center in the chicken's eye.

Isthmus: The part of the female reproductive tract where the inner and outer shell membranes are added.

J

Jake: A young male turkey.

Jejunum: A portion of the small intestine.

Jenny: A young female turkey.

K

Keel: The breast bone of birds.

Keet: A young (baby) guinea fowl.

Keratin: Key structural material of feathers (as well as wool, hooves, and human skin, hair and nails).

Knob: Protrusion from the skull.

L

Lacing: border of contrast color around the entire web of a feather.

Layer cycle: The period from the onset of lay until the natural moult causes a cessation of production. Usually used to describe the period during which an economic level of production is being maintained.

Layer: A female in lay. Usually used to refer to females kept solely for egg production for human consumption.

Lighting (artificial): The use of controlled artificial light to regulate the day length under which the stock are kept.

Litter: material scattered on the floor of a poultry house to absorb moisture and manure (also called bedding).

Liveability: The expression used to describe the number of survivors in a flock.

Lopped comb: A comb that falls to one side.

Lux: A unit of illumination equal to one lumen per square metre. Used to measure the brightness or intensity of light.

M

Magnum: The portion of the avian oviduct in which the thick white (albumen) is added.

Mandible: Upper or lower bony portion of the beak.

Mealy: Term used to describe plumage flecked with lighter color as if dusted with flour.

Mechanical transmission: Disease causing agents carried on a surface (such as shoes, tires, shovels, etc.).

Membrane: A thin, soft, pliable layer.

Metabolism: The physical and chemical processes that produce and maintain a living body.

Mite: A type of external parasite.

Molt (Moult): A part of the hen's reproductive cycle when she stops laying and loses her body feathers.

Morbidity: A health problem of a bird that typically requires it to be put down.

Mortality: Death due to disease or accident.

Mossy: Indistinct, irregular, or messy-looking markings that break up or destroy the intended color pattern on feathers.

Mottled: Plumage where a percentage of feathers are tipped with white; a discoloration of egg yolk caused by damage to the yolk membrane.

Mounting: When the rooster mates with a hen.

Muff: Fluffy feathers on the face of chickens (tufts are feathers that protrude from the face).

N

Necropsy: A postmortem (after death) examination of an animal (equivalent to a human autopsy).

Necrotic: Pertaining to dead tissue.

Nest egg: Artificial egg placed in a nest to encourage hens to lay there.

Nest run: Ungraded eggs.

O

Oil sac: Large oil gland on the back of birds at the base of the tail and used by the bird to preen or condition feathers (also called the uropygial or preen gland).

Osteomyelitis: Inflammation of the bone marrow.

Osteoporosis: Thinning and weakening of the bones.

Ova: Female germ cells that become eggs.

Ovary: A part of the female avian reproductive tract which holds the female genetic material and collects the yolk material normally associated with eggs.

Oviduct: A part of the female avian reproductive tract where the egg white (albumen), shell membranes, shell and bloom (cuticle) are added to form a complete egg.

Oviposition: The laying of an egg.

Ovulation: The release of a yolk from the ovary.

Ovum: The female germ cells in the ovary (plural = ova).

P

Pasting: Loose droppings sticking to the vent area.

Peachick: A young (baby) peafowl.

Peacock: An adult make peafowl.

Peahen: An adult female peafowl.

Pecking order: The social rank of individuals within a flock.

Peep: A term for chick sometimes used by small flock owners.

Pellets: A form of feed where the contents are compressed into bite-sized morsels.

Pendulous crop: A crop that is impacted and enlarged and hangs down in an abnormal manner.

Penicled: Crosswise lines or bars on feathers that form a pattern.

Perch: A place where chickens can get off the floor (also called a roost).

Perosis: Malformation of the hock joint.

Persistency of lay: The ability of a hen to lay eggs steadily over a long period of time.

Pick out: Vent damage caused by other chickens' pecking.

Pigeon milk: A cottage-cheese looking crop substance produced by both the male and female pigeon to feed the young from hatch till about 10 days of age.

Pigmentation: The color of a chicken's beak, shanks and vent.

Pin bones: Pubic bones.

Pin feathers: A developing feather on a bird.

Pip: When a chick breaks through the shell.

Pipping: Breaking through the shell prior to hatch.

Plumage: The total set of feathers covering a bird.

Post: To conduct a postmortem (after death) examination.

Poult: Young (baby) turkey or pheasant.

Poultry: A term for domestic fowl raised for meat, eggs, feathers, work or entertainment.

Preen gland: An oil sack on the back and near the base of the tail of birds providing oil used in preening (also called the oil or uropygial gland).

Preening: To straighten and clean feathers, typically with oil.

Prolapse: When there is vent damage, typically caused by laying an very large egg (also referred to as a blowout).

Proventriculus: The true stomach of birds where pepsin and acid are produced

Pubic bones: Two bones that end in front of the vent of birds.

Pullet: Immature female bird (used with several species of birds, but most commonly with chickens).

Purebred: Offspring from a hen and rooster of the same breed.

R

Rales: Any abnormal sounds coming from the airways of birds.

Ratite: A type of domestic bird that does not have a keel bone and includes ostriches, emus and rheas.

Render: The process by which slaughter by-product are treated to convert them into protein products for use in animal feeds.

Rigor mortis: Stiffness following death.

Roach back: Deformed, hunched back (a disqualification when showing poultry).

Roaster: A meat-type chicken raised to a size that makes them suitable for roasting.

Roost: A place where chickens can get off the floor (also called a perch).

Rooster: Adult male chicken (also referred to as a cock).

Rumpless: Genetic trait in some chicken breeds where they have no tail.

S

Saddle: a part of a bird's back just before the tail.

Sanitize: to clean and disinfect in order to kill germs.

Scales: small, hard, overlapping plates that cover a chicken's shanks and toes.

Scratch: the habit of chickens to scrape there claws against the ground to dig up food items; also a term used for any whole grains fed to chickens.

Sexed chicks: day-old chicks that are separated into separate groups of male and female chicks.

Sex feathers: rounded hackle, saddle, and tail feathers on a hen; pointed hackle, saddle and tail feathers on a rooster.

Sex-linked: an inherited factor linked to the sex chromosomes and used in developing specific crosses to make sexing day-old chicks easier.

Shaft: part of the feather where the barbs are attached.

Shank: the part of a bird's leg between the foot and the hock.

Shell gland: the portion of the female avian reproductive tract where the shell is added to the egg (also called the 'uterus').

Sickles: Long, curved tail feathers of some roosters.

Side sprig: projection from the side of a single comb (a disqualification when showing single-comb breeds of chickens).

Spent (as in a spent hen): a hen that is no longer laying eggs.

Spike: round extension found at the end of a rose comb.

Splayed legs: the legs are positioned such that the bird is unable to stand up (also called 'spraddle legs').

Spur: the sharp horny protrusion from the back of a bird's shank (typically larger in males than in fem ales).

Squab: A young (baby) pigeon that has not yet left the nest; also refers to pigeon meat since pigeons are usually marketed before they leave the nest.

Squeaker: a young pigeon still in the nest.

Squirrel tail: tail that has more than a 90 degree angle.

Snood: the flap of skin that hangs over the turkey's beak.

Starve-out: a chick that has not eaten.

Straight-run (chicks): day-old chicks that have not been sorted by sex (also called unsexed).

Strain: a group of birds within a variety of a breed that has been bred by one person or company for generations.

Stub: down on the shank or toe of a clean-legged chicken.

U

Testes: The male reproductive glands (located internally in birds).

Tin hen: Slang for an incubator.

Tom: an Adult male turkey (also referred to as a 'gobbler').

Torticollis: Twisted or wry neck.

Toxin: A poison produced by microorganisms.

Trio: A male with two females of the same species, breed and variety.

Type: The size and shape of a chicken that tells you what breed it is.

Unsexed: Day-old chicks that have not been sorted by sex (also called straight-run).

Urates: Uric acid (the avian form of pee).

Uropygial gland: Large oil gland on the back and at the base of the tail of birds providing oil for the birds to preen their feathers (also called the preen or oil gland).

V

Variety: Subdivision of a breed, according to plumage color, comb type, etc.

Vent: The common outside opening of the cloaca in birds through which the digestive, excretory and reproductive tracts empty

Verticle transmission: Disease transmitted from parent to offspring through hatching eggs

Vitelline membrane: The thin membrane that surrounds the yolk

Vulture hock: Feather-legged breeds where the feathers grow off the shank and touch the ground

W

Wattles: The flap of skin under the chin of a chicken or turkey

Web: The network of interlocking parts that give a feather its smooth appearance; a part of the feet of waterfowl

Wet-blub thermometer: A thermometer used to measure the amount of moisture or water vapor in the air (humidity).

Wing clipping: A procedure in which the primary wing feathers of one wing are cut to prevent flight.

Wry tail: Tail that lays to the left or gith side and is not symmetrical with the body line.

X

Xanthophylls: The yellow pigments found in leaves, grasses and green plants that are added as pigment to avian skin as well as providing the yellow color of egg yolks.

Y

Yolk sac: The membrane that surrounds the yolk in the incubating egg.

Yolk: The round yellow mass upon which the genetic material of the female (and male if the egg is fertilized) is located and that provides nutrients for the devloping embryo.

2

Taxonomy of Avian Species

Taxonomic classification of avian species is beyond the scope of this booklet. However, since the preliminary knowledge of bird species for students of avian medicine class is of interest, the following description of most common pet and wild birds are being attempted for their benefit.

GALLINEFORMES: This order includes domestic chicken, turkey, pheasants, peafowl, grouse, quail, guinea fowl, guans and curassows.

COLUMBIFORMES: Includes pigeons and doves.

PSITTACIFORMES: Includes parrots, which have strongly hooked maxilla with a flexible attachment to the skull. They also have dexterous zygodactyl feet (two digits point forward and two backwards). The order includes.

- **Large seed eating birds:** Macaw, parrot, cockatoo
- **Small seed eating birds:** Cockatiel, Budgerigar, Lovebird, and Lories.

STRUTHIONIFORMES: Includes Ostrich.

RHEIFORMES: Includes Rheas.

CASUARIFORMES: Includes Emu, Cassowaries.

APTERIGIFORMES: Includes Kiwis.

Ostrich, Rhea, Emu, Cassowaries, and Kiwi are collectively called RATITES. These are flightless birds. Although these belong to separate orders, each is closely related. These have reduced wing and weakly developed pectoral muscles. There are two toes in ostrich feet whereas others have three toes. The innermost two of cassowaries is armed with a long, sharp, dangerous claw. Ostrich, Rhea and EMU are found in open land, Cassowaries inhabit rain forests of New Guinea and Australia, and Kiwis live in forests of New Zealand. Kiwis have a long beak and eat earthworms and soil invertebrates. Others in the group are herbivorous.

FALCONIFORMES: Includes vultures, Falcons, Kites, Hawks and Eagles.

STRINGIFORMES: Owls.

Vulture, Falcons, Kites, Hawks, Eagles and Owls are collectively called RAPTORS. They are diurnal birds of prey. They have hooked beaks. Falcons have notched beak and large pointed wings. They dive or swoop on their prey at a great speed, striking with toes. Raptors prey on insects, birds, small mammals, reptiles and fish.

ANSERIFORMES: Includes ducks, geese and swan. They have blunt flatted beak and webbed feet with a hind toe. They feed aquatic vegetation, seeds and small invertebrates.

SPHENISCIFORMES: Includes Penguin.

PELECANIFORMES: Includes Pelican, Gannets etc.

CICONIIFORMES: Herons, Storks, Flamingos and Spoonbills.

PICIFORMES: Toucans, a popular cage bird.

PASSERIFORMES: Includes the largest number of bird species. Classified on their feeding habits:

a) **Insectivorous:** Barber, Flycatcher, and Shrike.

b) **Frugivorous:** Waxwing, Billbird

c) **Nectar feeders:** Sunbird, Honey creepers, Canary.

d) **Seed eaters:** Finches, Sparrows, Cardinals, and Goldfish.

e) **Omnivorous:** Corvid, Tanager, Starlings, Mynah, Oriole, Manakin, Bird of paradise, crows, and Jays.

Frequently kept pet birds.

Birds Frequently Kept as Pets

Psittacines	Passeriforms	Piciformes
Amazonparrot	Canary	Taucan
Budgerigar (parkeet, bugie)	Finch	
Caique parrot	Mynah	
Cockatiel		
Cockatoo		
Conure		
Lory		
Lovebird		
Macaw		
Parakeet		
Parrot		
Rosella		
Columbiformes	**Birds as prey**	**Miscellaneous**
Pigeons	Eagle	Turkey
	Hawk	Pheasant
	Kestrel	Fowl
	Falcon	Pea fowl
	Owl	Crane
		Dove

3

Immunity and Inflammation in Birds

Introduction

Anatomy of the immune system in birds differs from that in mammals. Immune cells are present in primary lymphoid organs (PLO) and secondary lymphoid organs (SLO). In birds, thymus and bursa of Fabricius (cloacal bursa) are primary lymphoid organs. Secondary lymphoid organs include the spleen, bone marrow, Harderian gland, aggregates of lymphoid tissue in various organs; i.e. in the gut called gut-associated lymphoid tissue (GALT); in bronchi called bronchial-associated lymphoid tissue (BALT). SLO contains aggregates of lymphocytes and antigen presenting cells. Birds do not have lymph nodes.

In PLO, the lymphoid cells are processed for differentiation and maturation. T lymphocytes differentiate and mature in the thymus, whereas B lymphocytes mature in bursa of Fabricius. Functional lymphocytes move from PLO to SLO. Like mammals, birds defend the body against pathogens through innate immunity (non-adaptive immunity) and adaptive or acquired immunity. Under innate immunity system, physical barriers present in birds play their important role preventing the entry of pathogens into the body. Physical barriers are feathers, skin, aggregates of lymphoid cells in various organs and ciliary defence in the respiratory system. Phagocytosis is first defence for pathogens entering the body, evading the physical barriers. Phagocytic cells include mainly heterophils and macrophages. Natural killer cells (NK cells), thrombocytes and complement also help in innate immunity.

Adaptive immunity is a particular defence which develops when the innate immunity is inadequate to impart protection. Adaptive immunity is antigen specific. T cell, B cell and macrophages play a major role in adaptive immunity. Adaptive immunity is brought about by antibodies (humoral immunity) or also by cells (cell-mediated).

Cell-mediated immunity is produced mainly by T cells. T cell recognises foreign antigen when antigen has been processed by antigen-presenting cells (APC) and complexed with major histocompatibility complex (MHC) molecules. MHC molecules are glycoprotein receptors coded by genes. Birds have a smaller number (19) of genes compared to humans (more than 200 genes). Most important APCs include macrophages, dendritic cells, and B cells. Based on surface molecules, T cells can be differentiated in CD4+ and CD8+. CD4+ is the T helper (T_H) lymphocyte. T_H (CD4+) cells recognise antigen when complexed with MHC II. After recognition of specific antigen, CD4+ cells are activated and initiate an immune response against the antigen. As in mammals, in chickens, antigens mediated by cytokines stimulate CD4+ (T_H) cells which differentiate into two separate populations: T_H1 and T_H2 helper cells. T_H1 are formed when a pathogen is intracellular in APCs. The primary function of T_H1 cells is stimulation and proliferation of CD4+. T_H2 cells help B lymphocytes to produce antigen specific antibodies. The known function of CD4+ is destruction through lysis of virus infected-cells.

Cytokines

Cytokines are small biologically active proteins secreted mainly by T cells, B cells, macrophages, and dendritic cells. The function of cytokines is to bind on the specific surface receptor of target cells and regulate immune response signalling between cells. Similar to mammals, production and function of cytokines in birds are same (interleukins, tumour necrosis factor).

Humoral Immunity

Humoral immunity is produced by secretion of immunoglobin (Ig) through B cells. B cells give rise to plasma cells which in turn produce antibodies. Ig (antibodies) is present mainly in blood. Small quantity may also be found in other body fluids. Antibodies react with pathogens (microorganisms) and cause their destruction. Important mechanisms through which antibodies work are: (1) Neutralizing antibodies bind and neutralise specific pathogens. It is mainly seen in virus-infected cells. Neutralized viruses are unable to attach to the surface receptors of target cells and replicate. (2) Opsonization. It covers the surface of pathogens (mainly bacteria) making them more prone to phagocytosis. (3) Complement. Pathogens activate production of complement. Complement destroys pathogens through cell membrane lysis system or phagocytosis.

Recognized types of antibodies in chickens are IgM, IgG and IgA. Similar to mammals, all three classes of antibodies have “heavy chain” and “light chain” polypeptide. However, the Ig molecules in birds are larger with a “switch region” between two polypeptides. The function of each class of antibodies is determined by a heavy chain. B cells use surface Ig to bind to antigens. Specific B cell population produces one type of light and heavy chain. To initiate Ig production antigen must react with B cell having homologous receptor. With the presence of a large variety of antigens, B cells need some mechanism to identify specific antigen. Numbers of genetic mechanisms occur during development of B cells, which help to attain needed diversity. In mammals, Ig diversity is achieved through gene rearrangement. Because of a small number of Ig genes in birds, gene diversity is obtained through gene conversion. B cells initially start producing IgM. As the immune response progresses, B cells switch to produce IgG and IgA, through a phenomenon "class switch". This class switch is influenced by various cytokines. IgG is usually produced after secondary vaccination. IgG is large antibody molecule compared to the mammalian counterpart. Because of the larger size of IgG in birds, it is also called IgY. IgA class of antibody in birds is involved in mucosal immunity. IgA in birds is found on the mucosal surfaces, some times in bile and a small quantity in the blood. An important function of IgA is the protection of mucosal surfaces from pathogens especially viruses.

Transfer of Immunity from Hens

Maternal transfer of immunity is a unique feature in avian species. Transfer of immunity from hens protects chicks from pathogens in the early phase of life. The duration of maternal immunity in chicks varies from 3 to 4 weeks.

The transfer mechanism from hen to chicks is interesting. The circulating Ig in the hen is deposited in the epithelial and glandular cells of the oviduct. From the oviduct, Ig is transferred to ovarian follicles and eventually stored in the yolk sac. Absorption of Ig from yolk starts around the 7th day of embryo development.

However, the peak of Ig is maximal during three days before hatch. This absorption continues for 1-2 days after hatch. IgM and IgA formed in the oviduct mucosa are also deposited in the albumen of the egg. Albumen diffuses into the amniotic fluid, and the embryo gets IgM and IgA by swallowing the amniotic fluid. Finally, the hatched chick has Ig in the blood and IgA and IgM in the intestines.

Inflammation in Birds

Mononuclear cells (monocytes and lymphocytes) are similar in mammals and birds. However, there is a significant difference within granulocytic series. Avian granulocyte heterophil corresponds to mammalian neutrophil. Heterophils in avian blood smears stained with Giemsa or Wright stain show basophilic nucleus with one or two lobes and deeply eosinophilic stained spindle shape cytoplasmic granules.

Experimental studies on avian inflammation showed that in acute inflammation there is an increase in heterophils (heterophilia) which peaks at 12 hours. Heterophilia, more pronounced between 12 and 24 hours, is accompanied by left shift and the presence of a vast number of immature cells. Immigration of heterophils in acute inflammation is the first line of defence. However, the influx of heterophils and monocytes within hours of an acute inflammatory process is a feature observed in many species of birds. The immigration events of heterophils and monocytes in the area of inflammation are similar to that in mammals. Like mammals, migration of leukocytes in birds is not dependent on vascular permeability.

Pathogenesis of acute inflammation in birds differs significantly from that of mammals. In mammals, accumulation of neutrophils in inflammation leads to liquefaction and abscess formation, which eventually resolves. In birds, on the other hand, necrotic heterophils are inspissated into a caseous mass rather than getting calcified. Eventually, a heterophilic granuloma is formed at the site of inflammation. Heterophilic granulomas comprise of dead heterophils in the centre surrounded by macrophages and occasionally foreign body giant cells. Heterophil granuloma lacks lymphocytes and plasma cells. Heterophil granuloma develops within a week of inflammation. A granuloma is surrounded by fibrous connective tissue. Heterophilic granulomas in birds are considered more defensive in isolating pathogens and irritants. Granulomas are advantageous except when they do not interfere with the function of the tissue. In birds, heterophils contain little or no hydrolytic enzyme activity. This absence of enzyme is considered the reason why exudate does not liquefy in birds.

Histiocytic granulomas in birds have similar etiological agents and have similar pathogenesis. Histiocytic granuloma develops mostly with intracytoplasmic pathogens. The absence of dead caseated heterophils in histiocytic granuloma is a differentiating feature between the two granulomas. In birds, calcification in histiocytic granuloma is usually not present.

Antimicrobial property of Heterophils

Heterophils are potent phagocytic cells of birds which readily phagocytose a variety of microbial agents. Similar to phagocytosis by neutrophils in mammals, complement, chemokines and cytokines assist the phagocytic activity of heterophils in birds.

Heterophils in birds have strong microbicidal power but unlike in mammal microbicidal activity of heterophils is not dependent on oxygen dependent killing of microbes. Upon phagocytosis of pathogens similar to neutrophils in mammals, heterophils also undergo respiratory burst, but production of hydrogen peroxide (H_2O_2) is very much low in heterophils. Heterophils also lack myeloperoxidase (MPO). Due to the absence of myeloperoxidase in heterophils, halogenation is not produced in birds. H_2O_2-MPO halide system is a very potent bactericidal system in neutrophils.

Non-oxidative microbicidal mechanism of heterophils is because of heterophil morphology. Heterophils consist of 2 types of granules in their cytoplasm. The larger granules contain cationic peptides, lysozymes and acid phosphatase. Peroxidase and alkaline phosphatase present in neutrophils are absent in heterophils. Cationic peptides present in larger granules of heterophils belong to the b-defensin class of antimicrobial peptides. These defensins differ from classical mammalian defensins. Defensins as a group are small cationic proteins that possess broad spectrum microbicidal property against bacteria, protozoa, fungi and enveloped viruses.

General responses to inflammation in mammals and birds are similar. In the pathogenesis of inflammation, birds mount both humoral and cellular reaction.

4

Avian Salmonellosis

Introduction

Avian salmonellosis is the term used to describe a large group of acute or chronic diseases caused by one or more members of the bacterial genus *Salmonella*, which is a member of the large family *Enterobacteriaceae*. Domestic poultry is known to constitute the largest single reservoir of Salmonella organism existing in nature. They include host specific and nonmotile members of the genus *S. enterica subspp. enterica pullorum/gallinarum*. If the infection of poultry is due to other *Salmonella* organisms other than *Salmonella enteric subspp. enterica gallinarum/pullorum*, the infection is then referred to as **paratyphoid.**

Pullorum/Gallinarum Disease/Fowl Typhoid

Etiology

Pullorum disease is caused by *Salmonella pullorum* and fowl typhoid by *Salmonella gallinarum.* Both bacteria have been grouped in a single serovar, *S. enterica* subsp. *enterica* serovar *Pullorum/gallinarum* of the family Enterobacteriaceae. Both members of the genus are non-motile. Both serovars have biochemical differences. Since epizootiology of the Pullorum and gallinarum is similar, they are described together for simplicity. *S. pullorum* and *S. gallinarum* possess the 'O' antigen 1, 9 and 12. Variation in antigen 12 has been described in *S. pullorum.*

Disease Occurrence

The disease is worldwide in distribution. However, in some countries, the disease has been successfully eradicated.

Hosts

Chickens and turkey are the natural hosts, the disease has been reported in many avian species, but the spread of the disease through infected ovaries has not been seen in species other than chicken and turkey.

Transmission

Transmission is mainly vertical through contaminated egg from infected birds. Egg gets contaminated following ovulation. The disease is also transmitted horizontally through faeces of reactor/infected birds. The relative Figure for vertical transmission with *S. pullorum* and *S. gallinarum* is unclear. However, this route of transmission is believed to be more with *S. pullorum.*

Transmission of *S. pullorum and S. gallinarum*

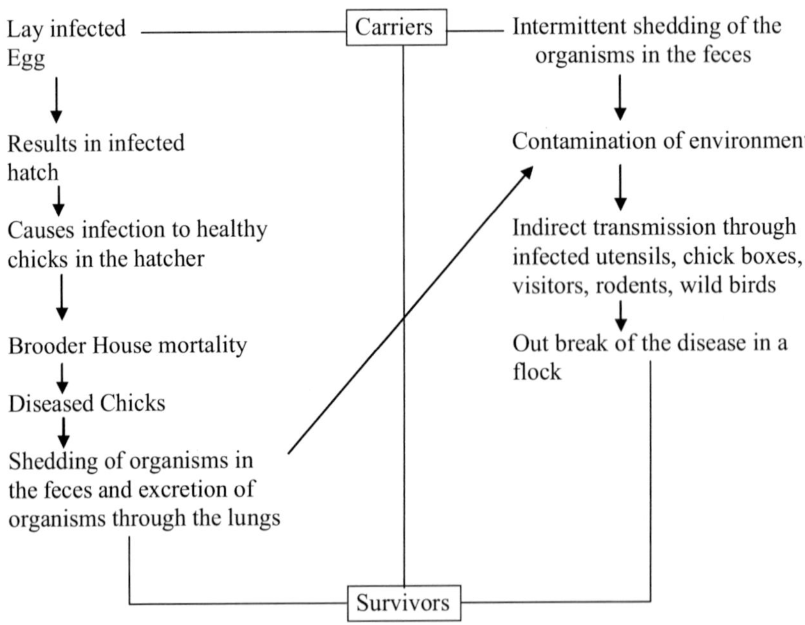

• Chicks

1) In the infected hatch, moribund and dead chicks are seen in the incubator. Many chicks die within a short time after hatching.
2) Chicks show weakness, loss of appetite and sudden death. Mortality starts on the 1st or 2nd day in the brooder house. In some cases, the peak of mortality is seen a week after. Mortality varies and in some cases may reach to 95%.
3) Some chicks show nervous signs like staggering and in-coordination of limbs; others show increased thirst and signs of respiratory distress. Some chicks appear sleepy with dropping wings and huddle close to the source of light and heat.

4) The most important sign is an accumulation of chalk white excreta, sometimes stained brown, around the vent.

5) A few chicks may show swelling of the limb joints.

6) The survivors show retarded growth and poor feathering. These survivors result in a high percentage of carriers at maturity.

• Adults

1) Adult flock does not show signs of an acute infection. The disease may spread in a flock for a longer period without clinical signs.

2) In rare cases when the disease is severe, the symptoms are similar to those of Fowl typhoid. In such cases, the first sign of the illness is general depression. The combs and visible mucous membranes are pale due to anaemia. There may be intermittent diarrhoea, and birds show fever. The disease continues for a week or longer with low mortality.

3) There is decreased egg production in the carrier flocks.

Mortality and Morbidity

Both vary from flock to flock, depending on the age, nutrition, and mode of exposure. In severe outbreaks, losses may be 100%. In vertically transmitted infection the maximum losses are during first two weeks.

Pathology

• Chicks

1) Low hatchability and increase in a number of piped embryos, (dead-in-shell).

2) There is omphalitis (inflammation of yolk sac). The yolk sac contents become watery and greenish yellow. Occasionally, yolk contents become cheesy in appearance and consistency.

3) The liver and spleen are enlarged, congested and may show small pinpoint to pinhead size necrotic foci (Figure 1) Kidneys show congestion and ureters filled with chalky white urates. Pericarditis may be observed in some chicks. A few chicks exhibit swelling of mainly hock joint, which contains yellow viscous fluid (Figure 2).

4) In chicks up to six week age, necrotic foci or nodules may be seen in heart muscles, (Figure 3) and abscesses in the lungs.

Adults

1) In chronic carriers, the lesions are found in the ovary of the hen. Lesions consist of misshapen ovules, or pedunculated ovules (Figure 4). The diseased ova usually contain oily and cheesy material enclosed in a thickened capsule. The pedunculated ova are attached to ovary by a stalk. Occasionally, the diseased ova detach and fall into the abdominal cavity and produce extensive peritonitis and adhesions of abdominal viscera.

2) Lesions in adults dying of acute infection have enlarged liver with small necrotic foci (Figure 5). The liver takes bronze colour after exposure to air. Spleen and kidneys are swollen and congested.

Diagnosis

Although the history of disease on the premises, the symptoms and lesions may be suggestive of Pullorum disease and fowl typhoid, a final diagnosis must depend upon the isolation and identification of the organism. Specimens required for isolation of the bacteria:

1. In acute infections, the liver is preferred organ for culture.
2. In chronic infections, organisms can be isolated from the ovaries but not regularly. For more accuracy heart, liver, spleen, ovary and oviduct be cultured.

Differential Diagnosis

- Abscesses in the lung occasionally caused by *S. pullorum* and *S. gallinarum* may confuse with lesion caused by Aspergillus fungus or other fungi. Abscesses caused by fungi are more extensive involving bronchi, trachea and air sacs. Impression smears from the lesions stained for fungus can confirm the diagnosis.
- Localized lesions in joints and tendon sheaths caused by *S. pullorum* or *S. gallinarum* may be confused with other diseases causing joint infections. The condition should be differentiated from Mycoplasmosis, viral arthritis, chronic fowl cholera and deficiency of mineral and vitamins.
- Acute outbreaks of *S. pullorum* and *S. gallinarum* may be confused with other septicemic diseases like Fowl cholera, Staphylococcosis and Colibacillosis. Blood or tissue smears, stained with Grams stain are examined for the bacteria to make a tentative diagnosis.
- White nodular lesions in heart sometimes produced in young chicks with *S. pullorum* and *S. gallinarum* resemble tumours of Marek's disease. Histological examination of nodules is helpful in differential diagnosis.

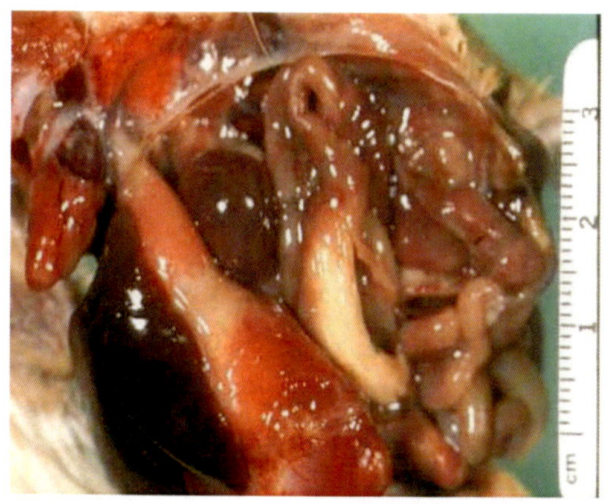

Fig. 1: *S. Pullorum/gallinarum* in 18 day-old chick (liver and spleen enlarged and congested, white cast in the cecum);

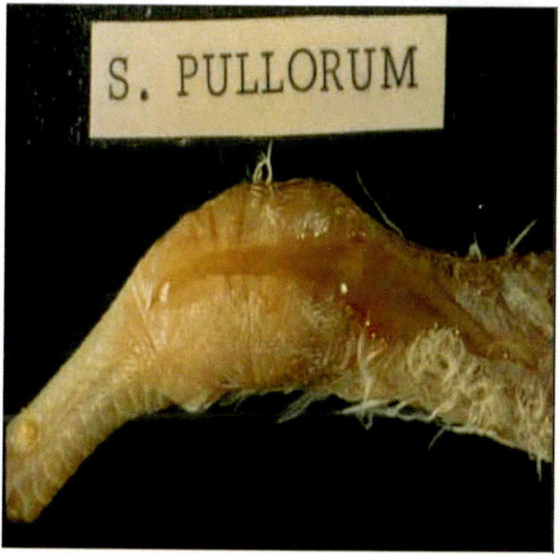

Fig. 2: *S. Pullorum/gallinarum* (hock joint synovitis)

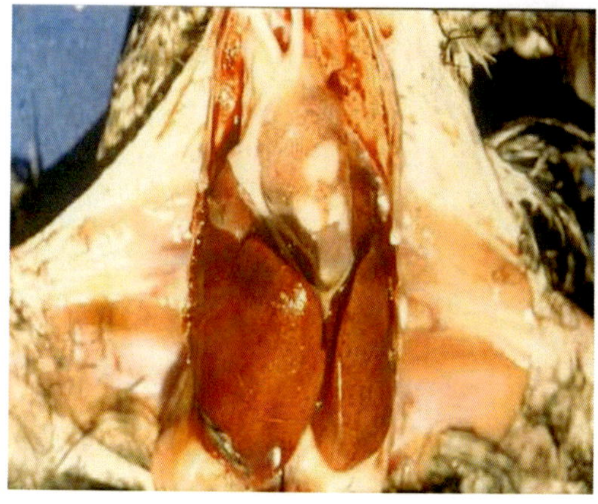

Fig. 3: *S. Pullorum/gallinarum*; 5 wk-old-chick (3 white nodules resembling tumors in the heart. Liver enlarged and congested).

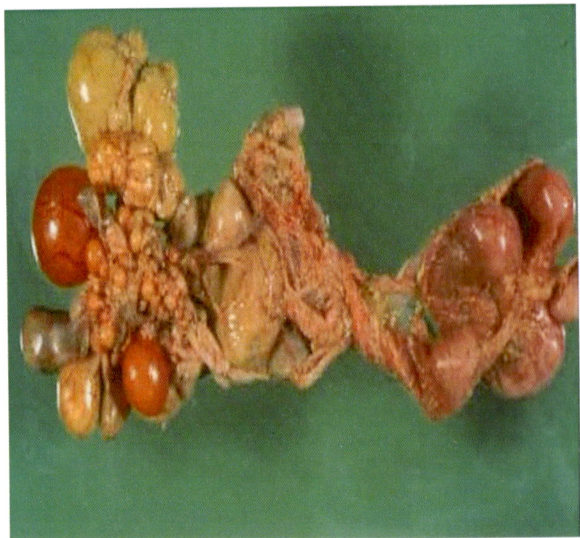

Fig . 4: *S. Pullorum/gallinarum;* Adult chicken (ovary with many misshapen nodular gray to yellow follicles)

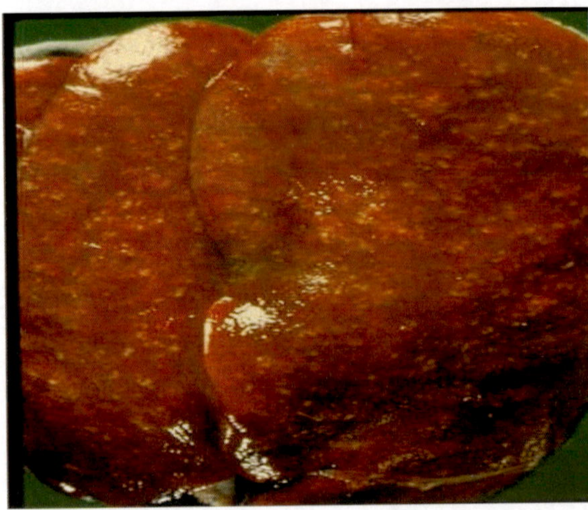

Fig. 5: *S. Pullorun/gallinarum* in adult chicken (enlarged liver with multifocal necrosis)

Treatment

Reasonably effective drugs are available for the treatment of Pullorum disease and fowl typhoid outbreaks. Sulfa drugs - sulfadiazine, sulfamerazine; antibiotics - tetracycline, ampicillin, spectinomycin, amoxycillin, flumequine and doxycycline were found to be effective.

Prevention and Control

Chickens and turkey flocks can be developed and maintained free of Pullorum disease and fowl typhoid. It could be achieved by hatching and breeding of poultry from *Salmonella pullorum and S. gallinarum* free breeding birds and by avoiding indirect and direct transmission of infection. Prevention and control can be practised by the following three ways:

1. **Elimination of carriers:** This is done by testing the birds for the presence of antibodies against *S. pullorum/ gallinarum*. Bird positive for antibodies is called, "reactor". The following methods have been described for testing:

   a) whole blood plate test (rapid whole blood plate test, RBPT)

   b) standard tube agglutination test

   c) rapid serum test

   d) micro-agglutination test

   RBPT is accepted for chickens and other methods used in turkeys, and other avian species.

2. **Management procedures:** General management practices and strict biosecurity at the farm to prevent the introduction of infection must be carried out.

3. **Incubator and hatchery hygiene:** Incubator and hatchery equipment be cleaned and disinfected after each batch of the hatch.

Vaccination

A live attenuated vaccine developed from a rough strain of *S. gallinarum* (AR) is used at 9 -10 weeks of age given subcutaneously preferably under the skin of the breast. In birds younger than eight weeks, vaccination may cause mortality.

Immunity lasts for 8-9 months. It reduces mortality of Fowl typhoid. The vaccine is advisable in commercial layer flocks where a disease is endemic. Breeder flocks should not be vaccinated, as antibodies produced after vaccination interferes with blood testing of the flock. Annual immunisation is recommended.

Antibiotics, particularly nitrofurans should not be used seven days before and fourteen days after administration of the vaccine. Do not repeat the vaccine within six months of the previous inoculation.

5

Paratyphoid Infections

Introduction

Disease caused by motile Salmonella species in birds is called "Paratyphoid infections". Paratyphoid infections are present in all parts of the world.

Etiology

Salmonella enterica includes six subspecies. Only one of that subspecies; *S. enteric subspecies enterica* includes more than 2500 motile serotypes.

Economic Importance

1. Paratyphoid infections are important bacterial diseases of hatching industry. Fertility and hatchability and egg production are affected. There is high mortality in young birds, and the survivors are stunted and weak.
2. Most of the bacteria included in this group are found pathogenic to other species of domestic animals and man. Hence, the group forms a serious public health problem.

Hosts of Paratyphoid Infections

In domestic poultry: turkeys and chickens. Outbreaks of the disease have also been recorded in geese, ducks and pigeons. In pet birds: it has been reported in many including finches, budgerigars, canaries, cockatiels, macaws, pigeons and Amazon parrots.

They are a common pathogen of cattle, swine, sheep, goat, dog, horse, fox, rabbit, etc. In animals mortality due to paratyphoid organisms usually occur in young and old weak animals. Animals are mostly healthy carriers and shed the organisms in their faeces. Humans get infected with most of the paratyphoid organisms, recovered from poultry. In man, they produce septicemia and lesions of gastroenteritis.

Transmission

There are many ways of transmission.

- **Through the Egg:** It is an important route of transmission.

  1) **Direct Ovarian Transmission:** In ducks, geese & pigeons and turkeys the organisms localises in ovaries and transmitted directly through ovaries. In chickens, the ovarian transmission is reported in *S. enterica subspecies enterica serovar Enteritidis* The frequency of ovarian transmission for other organisms of this group is unknown.

  2) **Egg Shell Contamination and Penetration:** Paratyphoid organisms mostly localise in the intestine and gall bladder of the hosts. They are eliminated intermittently in faeces and thus contaminate egg shell, feed and water. Fecal contamination of eggshell during the process of laying is most important. As the egg passes through the cloaca, Salmonella in faeces attach to the warm wet surface of the shell and may be drawn inside as it cools. After the egg has been laid, it may also get contaminated with nests or floor.

     a) In the brooder house, it is transmitted through contaminated water, and feed.

     b) **Mice, rats and wild birds** sometimes act as mechanical carriers and spread infection.

     c) **Cattle,** sheep, **goat, swine, rabbit, dog and cat** are a good source of infection to poultry. **The man may also act as a source of infection.**

     d) **Man gets infected** by consuming contaminated egg and poultry meat and also by handling contaminated poultry products.

Symptoms

1) The symptoms of paratyphoid are similar to those observed in Pullorum disease and Fowl Typhoid.

2) A high number of piped and dead embryos are found in the incubator.

3) In brooder house outbreaks the chicks stand with head lowered, eyes closed, wings drooping and feathers ruffled. There is watery diarrhoea with pasty vents. The birds huddle together towards the source of the heat.

4) Adult birds do not show outward signs of the infection. They are chronic carriers of the organisms in the intestinal wall.

5) In growing birds, the symptoms of the disease include loss of appetite, diarrhoea and dehydration.

Gross Lesions

1) In peracute outbreaks, the lesions may be completely absent.
2) In incubator and brooder house mortalities, the most constant lesions include omphalitis with coagulated yolk, hemorrhagic liver and spleen with pinpoint foci, congested kidneys and pericarditis.
3) In an acute outbreak, in growing and adult birds, lesions include congested and swollen liver, hemorrhagic spleen and kidneys, necrotic enteritis, pericarditis and peritonitis.

Diagnosis

1) History, clinical signs and postmortem lesions may be suggestive of paratyphoid infection. However, the final diagnosis depends on the isolation and identification of the organism.
2) Isolation of the organism can be made from the visceral organs of birds that have died of infection. The yolk sac and its contents are the best sources for culture from embryos. The shell and shell membranes are cultured from the hatching eggs.
3) Birds, which survive an outbreak and become carriers may excrete the organisms intermittently in their faeces for several weeks or a few months. Hence examination of many faecal swab is necessary from such birds.
4) From duck, turkey, goose and pigeon ovaries are the best sample for culture.
5) Samples from the feed can be cultured for isolation.

Serological Testing

The tube agglutination test can be used for the detection of adult carrier birds. But it is essential to know which serotype is present and use appropriate antigens for the test. It is important to have both "O" and "H" antigen components, since at a particular time antibody to either "O" or "H" antigen may be present. Paratyphoid infections have never been successfully tested by RBPT because of the low level of antibodies produced by paratyphoid organisms.

Treatment

It is similar to that described for Pullorum disease and Fowl typhoid.

Prevention and Control

Since faecal contamination of eggs by chronic carriers is the primary source of infection to the incubator and brooder; the hatchery and flock sanitation is the most important in the prevention and control of paratyphoid infection of poultry.

Elimination of carriers from breeding flock not possible because of the following reasons

1) Paratyphoid organisms are usually restricted to the intestinal tract, and infected birds give rise to intermittent positive reaction to agglutination test. Moreover, because of "O" and "H" antigens, the antibody titer is variable from test to test.

2) Intestinal excretion of microorganisms is usual. It makes the litter infected even after removal of reactors at one test, and further carriers are produced as a result of re-infection. Because of these reasons the serological test is not usually practised on a large scale to eliminate the infection. However, breeder flocks should be monitored bacteriologically for paratyphoid organisms through screening the incubator mortality/dead embryos.

Vaccination

There are no vaccines for paratyphoid organisms. However, a variety of vaccines is now available for control of *S. Enteritidis*. Many countries are using the vaccine with promising results. Since *S. Enteritidis* and *S. pullorum/ gallinarum* are antigenically related, birds vaccinated with *S. Enteritidis* could show a positive reaction to *S. pullorum* antigen.

6

Arizonosis

S. enterica subspecies arizonae (Salmonella arizonae), the cause of an acute septicemic disease in young turkey poults.

Host Range

S. arizonae are reported from a variety of avian, mammalian and reptile species. Among avian in addition to turkeys, it has been reported in **chicks, ducklings, psittacines and passerines.**

Transmission

Organism is present in the intestinal tract of infected birds. Hence transmission is similar to motile salmonellae. Many workers have reported transmission in turkeys through infected ovaries. Wild birds, reptiles, rats and mice are reported as the common reservoir of the organism. The organism is also transmitted by direct contact and through contaminated feed and water.

Clinical Signs

A. Poults and chicks

1) Listlessness, diarrhoea, leg-weakness, twisting of the neck and pasting around the vent.

2) Poults and chicks huddle together and sit on hocks (Figure 6).

3) They may develop blindness because of caseous material covering the retina.

4) A few poults may show nervous signs in severe outbreaks.

5) There is high mortality reaching 50%. Mortality continues up to 3-4weeks.

B. Adults do not show clinical signs and mortality.

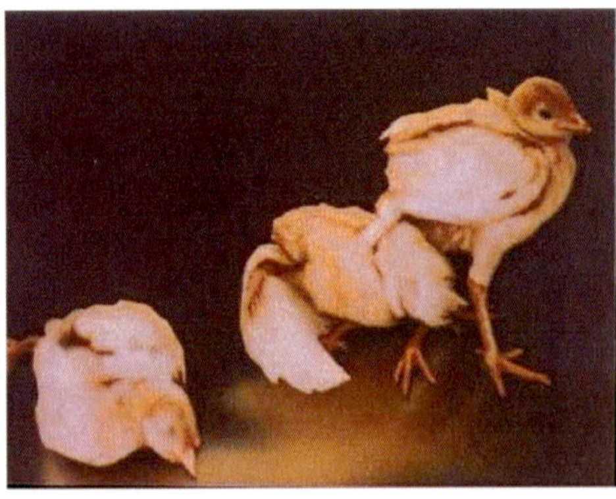

Fig. 6: *S. Arizona* infection in turkey poults with clinical signs of weakness and tendency to sit on hocks

Lesions

Lesions are similar to paratyphoid infections. In addition to micro- necrosed liver, caseous exudate in the abdominal cavity, and distended heart; most frequent finding is exudate in the vitreous of eyeballs. Severe meningitis has also been reported.

Diagnosis

High mortality, nervous signs and blindness in turkey poults are suggestive of *arozonosis*.

Differential Diagnosis

1) Nervous signs- Newcastle disease, Aspergillosis, Vitamin E deficiency.
2) Blindness- Aspergillosis.
3) Isolation and identification of the organism confirm the diagnosis.
4) Serology is helpful in diagnosis.

Treatment

Furazolidone in feed or water and injectable gentamicin and spectinomycin are permitted for use. These drugs reduce the mortality and spread of infection but do not eliminate carriers. Hygienic procedures for egg collection and treatment of eggs before incubation gives promising results.

Prevention and Control

- Similar to motile Salmonella.

Immunization

Many combinations of bacterins are being tried, but until now no effective vaccine is available.

7

Avian Mycoplasmosis

Introduction

From avian species alone approximately 20 mycoplasma serotypes have been isolated and characterised. Out of them, three serotypes (*M. gallisepticum, M. meleagridis* and *M. synoviae*) are most typical and pathogenic. A serotype *M. iowae* causes low hatchability in turkeys. Mycoplasmas are bacteria that lack cell wall and belong to the class Mollicutes. Although they have been considered extracellular agents, scientists admit nowadays that some of them are obligatory intracellular microorganisms, whereas all other mycoplasmas are considered facultative intracellular organisms

MYCOPLASMA GALLISEPTICUM

(Chronic Respiratory Disease (CRD), Air sac disease or Air sacculitis)

M. gallisepticum causes chronic respiratory disease (CRD) in chickens and infectious sinusitis of turkeys. Chronic respiratory disease in chickens also called "air sac disease or air sacculitis" refers to complicated, *Mycoplasma gallisepticum* (MG) infection with some respiratory viruses and *E. coli* infection. The disease is worldwide in distribution.

Hosts

M. gallisepticum causes disease in chickens and turkeys. However, *M. gallisepticum* has been isolated from many species of domestic birds, pet birds, wild and free flying birds.

Transmission

Transmission takes place in two ways:

1) **Direct Contact:** It spreads by air borne dust or droplet from the infected carrier chickens.

2) **Through the Egg:** Infection is also transmitted through the egg in chickens and turkeys. Egg gets infected while passing through the oviduct.

Clinical Signs

The incubation period is variable depending on age, the rate of exposure and concomitant infections by respiratory viruses and bacteria. The disease is more severe in winter months than the summer.

In Broilers

1) The outbreaks occur between 4 to 8 weeks of age.
2) In uncomplicated cases, morbidity is very high, but mortality is low.
3) Most of the infected broiler flocks show clinical signs of complicated CRD (air sac disease). In such flocks, mortality may rise to 30-35%.
4) Swelling of nasal sinuses and occasional coughing is noticed.
5) The birds show retarded growth and downgrading of the carcass.

In adult chickens

1) Clinical signs usually develop near the onset of egg production.
2) Tracheal rales, nasal discharge and coughing are the main clinical signs.
3) Feed consumption is reduced, and birds lose weight.
4) In laying flock, the egg production is at a lower level.

Gross Lesions in Chickens

1) Catarrhal exudate is present in nasal, paranasal passages, trachea, bronchi and air sacs.
2) In uncomplicated CRD, air sac membranes show small pinpoint to pinhead size greyish beads representing lymphofollicular aggregates seen under the microscope.
3) In complicated field cases, the air sacs contain caseous pus, (Figure 7 & 8) and have lesions of fibrinous or fibrinopurulent pericarditis and perihepatitis (Figure 9). (refer *E. coli* chapter).
4) Lungs show congestion and pneumonic patches.

In turkeys

Clinical signs and gross lesions of infectious sinusitis

1) Like chickens, clinical signs usually develop near maturity.
2) The main clinical sign is swelling of the head because of inflammation in the infraorbital sinus (Figure 10). Swelling may be unilateral or bilateral. The condition is seen for longer periods of time in untreated cases.
3) The turkeys lose weight causing the downgrading of the carcass.

Diagnosis

Although clinical signs and gross lesions are suggestive of *M. gallisepticum* infection, isolation and identification of organisms do confirmation. Isolation can be done on artificial media using trachea, air sacs or exudate as inoculum. Isolation of organism can also be made in 7 -days old embryonated chicken egg.

The following serological procedures available for MG diagnosis may be an added advantage in confirmation of the diagnosis:

a) Tube agglutination test
b) Rapid serum plate agglutination test
c) Hemagglutination inhibition test
d) Fluorescent antibody test
e) Agar gel precipitation test
f) ELISA test
g) PCR-based procedures

Differential Diagnosis

1) **Chickens**: Infectious coryza usually has similar clinical signs. They can be differentiated by cultural examination.
2) **Turkeys:** Fowl cholera, ornithosis, and turkey coryza might pose a problem of diagnosis. These should be distinguished by specific cultural and serological tests.

Treatment

Various antibiotics and chemicals namely streptomycin, chlortetracycline, oxytetracycline, erythromycin, spiramycin and tylosin have been used in feed or drinking water or injections for the treatment. Out of all, tylosin has been the drug of choice. It is used either as subcutaneous injection 8-10 mg per kg body weight or given at the rate of 0.5g/litre of drinking water for 3-5 days. Tiamulin and Baytril are other good drugs being used recently.

Prevention and Control

1. Immunization: Suitable vaccines are not available which give 100 percent protection. However, inactivated MG bacterins and live culture vaccines are being used in commercial laying flocks with variable results.
2. Medication of breeders
3. Egg dipping in antibiotics before incubation
4. Management procedures

MYCOPLASMA MELEAGRIDIS

M. meleagridis is specific bacteria affecting turkeys. It is egg transmitted disease, and the lesions are mainly seen in the progeny hatched from infected hens.

Host

Turkeys are natural hosts. Chickens are not infected by *M. meleagridis*

Transmission

It is transmitted mainly through the eggs. Direct and indirect transmission also occurs.

Clinical Signs and Lesions

1) Turkey poults show lesions of air sacculitis at one day of age just after the hatch. However, no respiratory signs are seen. In some infected hatch, lesions develop later in 3-5 weeks.
2) Lesions of air sacculitis are mostly in the thoracic air sacs, extending to abdominal air sacs 2-3 weeks later.
3) There are associated skeletal lesions, which include twisting and shortening of the tarsometatarsus bone (Figure 11), swelling of hock joints (Figure 12) and deformation of cervical vertebrae. Skeletal lesions are mostly seen in 1-6 week old poults.
4) The egg production and fertility in the infected flock is not affected. However, there is 4% to 5% mortality of embryos in the late incubation period.

Diagnosis

1) Air sac lesions in day old poults are suggestive.
2) Isolation and identification of the organism can confirm the diagnosis.
3) Serological tests as used for *M. gallisepticum* are effective in diagnosis.

Differential Diagnosis

Skeletal abnormalities may be differentiated from the nutritional deficiency of minerals.

Treatment

It is similar to that described for *M. gallisepticum* .

Prevention and Control

Vaccines are not available for *M. meliagridis.* Because most of the turkey hens get infected through contaminated semen, care should be taken to avoid such infection. Other methods of control are similar to those described for *M. gallisepticum*.

MYCOPLASMA SYNOVIAE

Mycoplasma synoviae infects chickens, turkeys and guinea fowl. *M. synoviae* isolates are differ significantly in their pathogenicity. Two major manifestations of infection are seen.

1) It produces primarily exudative synovitis, tenosynovitis and bursitis.
2) It causes sub-clinical infection of the upper respiratory tract, and when complicated by Newcastle disease virus or Infectious bronchitis virus it produces air sac lesions.

Transmission

It is similar to that described for *M. gallisepticum.*

Clinical Signs

1) The disease appears in the second week in chicks infected by egg transmission. The incubation period is 2-3 weeks in contact exposed chickens.
2) Clinical signs are seen between 4-16 weeks in chickens and between 10-24 weeks in turkeys. The affected birds show pale comb, lameness, ruffled feathers and retarded growth.

3) There is swelling around the joints. Any joint of the body may be involved, but hock joint and footpads are involved (Figure 13, 14). The birds remain active and feed and drink well even with severe joint lesions.

4) Respiratory tract infection may be asymptomatic or only slight rales are present.

Gross Lesions

1) Lesions start with the presence of viscous creamy to grey exudate in the synovial membranes of joints and tendon sheaths. In late stages of the disease, the exudate becomes caseous.

2) In some birds, caseous exudate may be found over the skull and along the neck extending into the air sacs.

3) In approximately half of the number of the infected birds, the liver and spleen are enlarged, mottled and greenish to dark red. Kidneys are swollen and pale.

Diagnosis

1) Pale comb, emaciation, lameness and enlarged hock joint and footpad may give a presumptive diagnosis.

2) The diseases can be confirmed by isolation and identification of *M. synoviae*. Primary isolation is done in 5-7 days old embryonated chicken egg via yolk sac inoculation.

3) Inoculation of Susceptible Host: 0.25 ml of the yolk from infected embryos or joint exudate from natural cases may be inoculated into foot pad of two week old chicken. Typical lesions of synovitis develop in 4-10 days.

4) Serological methods: Plate test can be done similar to *M. gallisepticum*. The antigen is commercially available. Other tests used are:

   a. Tube agglutination test

   b. Hemagglutination inhibition test (HI)

   c. Agar gel precipitation test

   d. Fluorescent antibody test.

   e. PCR- based methods

Cross-reaction with *M. gallisepticum* occurs but less common in HI and tube agglutination tests.

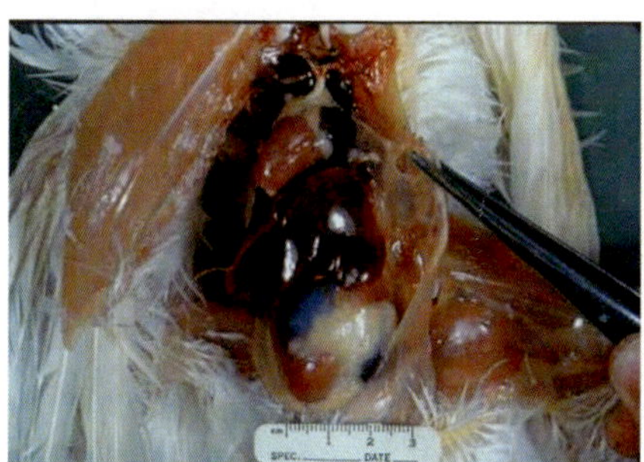

Fig.7: Chicken. Air saculitis seen as thickened air sac membrane.

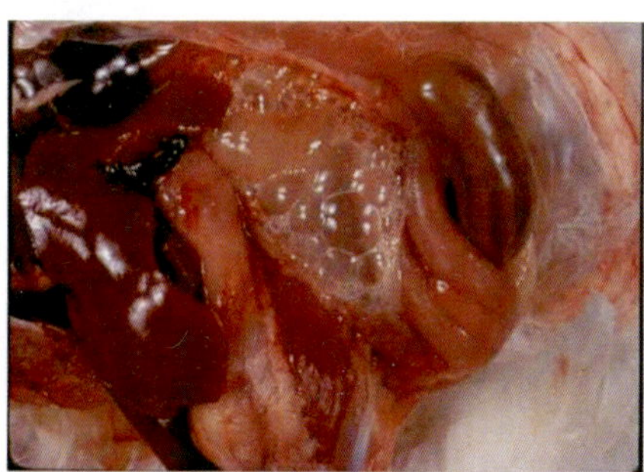

Fig. 8: Chicken. Lesions of air saculitis in abdominal air sac

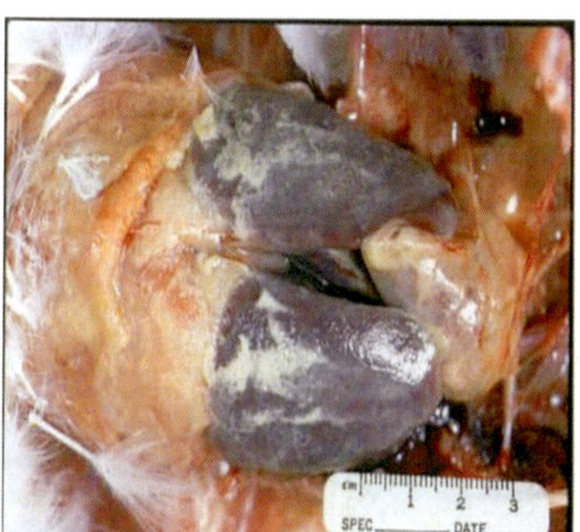

Fig. 9: Complicated *Mycoplasma gallisepticum* infection (pericarditis and perihepatitis)

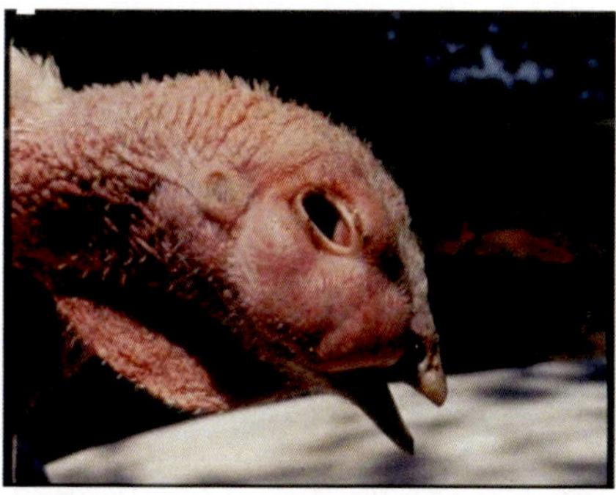

Fig. 10: *Mycoplasma gallisepticum* in turkey (swollen sinuses- infectious sinusitis)

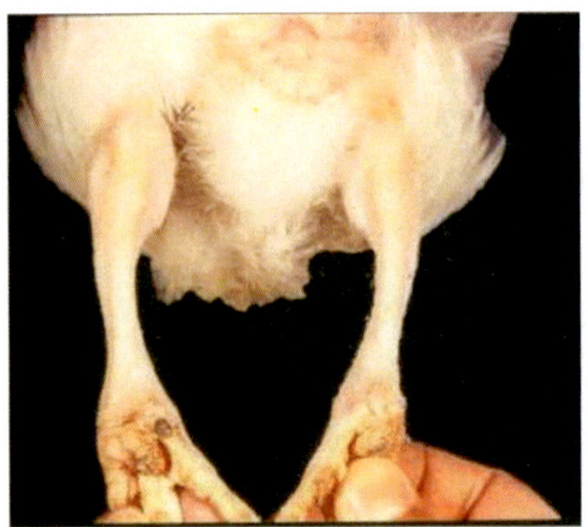

Fig. 11: *M. meleagridis*; 3-wk-old turkey poult with bowing of tarso-metatarsal bone.

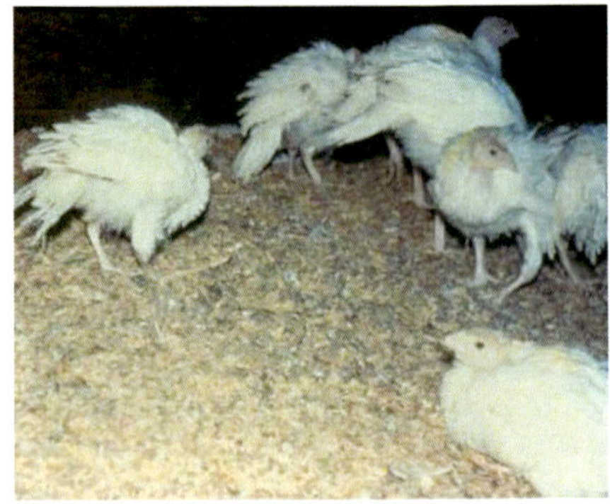

Fig.12: 10-wks-old turkey poults with swelling of hock joint infected with *M. meleagridis*.

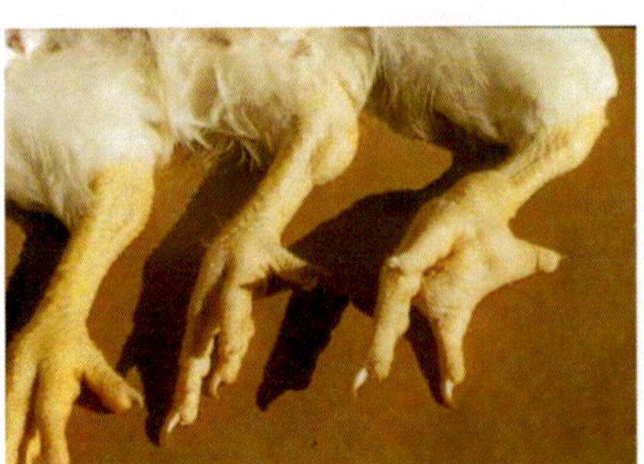

Fig. 13: *Mycoplasma synoviae* infection typical lesion- swollen foot pads.

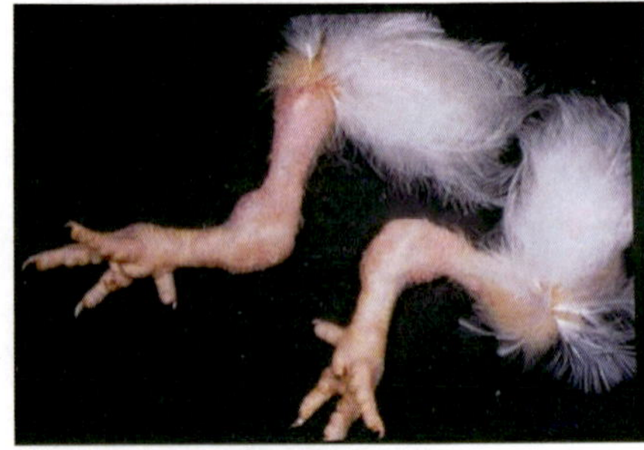

Fig. 14: Swollen hock and foot pads in MS infection.

Treatment

Chlortetracycline at the rate of 200g per ton of feed for 10-14 days controls the disease. For prevention, this medicine has been used at a half dose level, but it needs to be given continually.

Prevention and Control

Similar to that described for *M. gallisepticum.*

Vaccination

An inactivated, oil-emulsion bacterin is commercially available, but its efficacy has not yet been proved.

8

Colibacillosis / *Escherichia Coli* Infections

Introduction

Escherichia coli (E. coli) infections are responsible for significant economic losses to the poultry industry, worldwide. Disease conditions caused purely or partly by *E. coli* are as under:

1) Early embryonic mortality and chick mortality.
2) Coli septicemia and air sac disease.
3) Other disease conditions associated with *E. coli* are:
    a. Coli granuloma
    b. Peritonitis and Salpingitis
    c. Synovitis
    d. Ophthalmitis
    e. Pericarditis
    f. Swollen head syndrome
    g. Avian cellulitis
    h. Coli septicemia of ducks

E. coli infection is mostly reported in chickens, turkeys and ducks, however, it infects most mammals and birds. Pathogenic and nonpathogenic strains of *E. coli* are commonly present in the intestinal tract. Pathogenic strains can not be differentiated from non-pathogenic strains by only morphological characters and biochemical tests. Pathogenicity tests have to be done to identify the pathogenic strains.

A. Early embryo mortality and chick mortality

1) Fecal contamination of eggs is the most important source of infection similar to paratyphoid organisms. Other sources of infection to egg may be through ovary or oviduct.
2) The bacteria (*E. coli*) multiply in the yolk sac causing the death of embryo usually in the late incubation period. In the majority of the infected hatch, the mortality continues up to three weeks.
3) Chicks dying during the first week show lesions of omphalitis and peritonitis. Changing of yolk contents from viscid yellow to watery yellow brown or yellow green or caseous marks "Omphalitis".
4) In some cases, there may be no embryonic or chick mortality, and only signs of the disease observed are retained yolk sac and reduced weight gain.
5) Stress factors like low brooding temperature, fasting of the chicks, and stress during transport increase the incidence of chick mortality in case of E. coli infection.

Transmission of *Escherichia Coli*

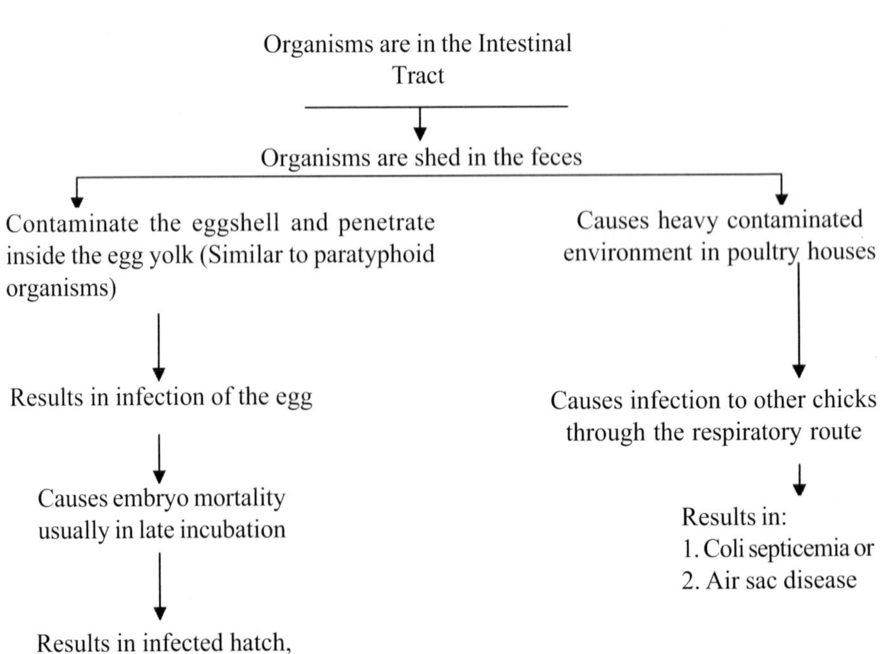

B. Early embryo mortality and chick mortality

1) Fecal contamination of eggs is the most important source of infection similar to paratyphoid organisms. Other sources of infection to egg may be through ovary or oviduct.

2) The bacteria (*E. coli*) multiply in the yolk sac causing the death of embryo usually in the late incubation period. In the majority of the infected hatch, the mortality continues up to three weeks.

3) Chicks dying during the first week show lesions of omphalitis and peritonitis. Changing of yolk contents from viscid yellow to watery yellow brown or yellow green or caseous marks "Omphalitis".

4) In some cases, there may be no embryonic or chick mortality, and only signs of the disease observed are retained yolk sac and reduced weigh t gain.

5) Stress factors like low brooding temperature, fasting of the chicks, and stress during transport increase the incidence of chick mortality in case of E. coli infection.

A. Coli septicemia/air sac disease

The disease occurs most frequently in broiler chicken, between 3 and 12 weeks age, but the maximum incidence is at 6-9 weeks. The frequency of the disease has increased with intensive methods of broiler production. It is common in overcrowded flocks. The route of infection seems to be respiratory tract. Although, *E. coli* organisms are usually present in the intestinal tract, the onset of coli septicemia/ air sac disease result from the inhalation of dust contaminated with *E. coli*. A variety of predisposing factors, other than intensive methods of poultry rearing, may be of importance in the pathogenesis of Colisepticemia/ air sac disease. Various combinations of mycoplasma and respiratory viruses such as infectious bronchitis virus and Newcastle disease virus make the respiratory route more susceptible to *E. coli* infection. Also, general debility caused by diseases such as coccidiosis, or by malnutrition or certain other viral infections like the infectious bursal disease, make the chicken more susceptible to *E. coli* infection.

Clinical Signs and Gross Lesions

1. Acute septicemic infection (Coli septicemia)

1) Mortality may be high, occasionally reaching more than 20%.

2) The lesions are mostly in the liver and heart. The liver is swollen and may have small pinhead necrotic foci. It is accompanied with pericarditis.

(Figure 15). The pericardial sac becomes cloudy, and epicardium is covered with light colour exudate. In some cases, the pericardial sac contains light yellow colour fibrinous exudate.

3) The spleen is enlarged and congested.

4) Necrotic eye lesions are sometimes seen with *E. coli* septicemia.

5) Pectoral muscles are occasionally seen congested.

2. Air sac disease

1) Mortality is mostly below 10%. However, morbidity is very high.

2) The birds are debilitated and show poor feed conversion. They are retarded in growth, and the carcass quality is poor.

3) The primary lesions are in the air sac. The air sac membranes become cloudy and later thickened. Caseous exudate is found on the respiratory surface of the air sacs.

4) The liver is swollen, dark in colour and show changes of perihepatitis. Often a false membrane covers the surface of the liver.

5) There are lesions of chronic pericarditis (Figure 16).

Other disease conditions/ Lesions caused by *E.coli*

1. Salpingitis and peritonitis

In laying hens when infection reaches abdominal air sac, it develops into chronic salpingitis. The size of caseous exudate may increase with time and block the oviduct.

2. Panophthalmitis

An unusual manifestation of *E. coli* septicemia. Usually one eye is affected. Microscopically, heterophils, mononuclear cells, and occasionally giant cells infiltrate around the necrosed eye tissue. Retina is mostly destroyed.

3. Synovitis

In acute septicemic form many birds develop synovitis. Many recover in a week but others may become chronic and emaciated.

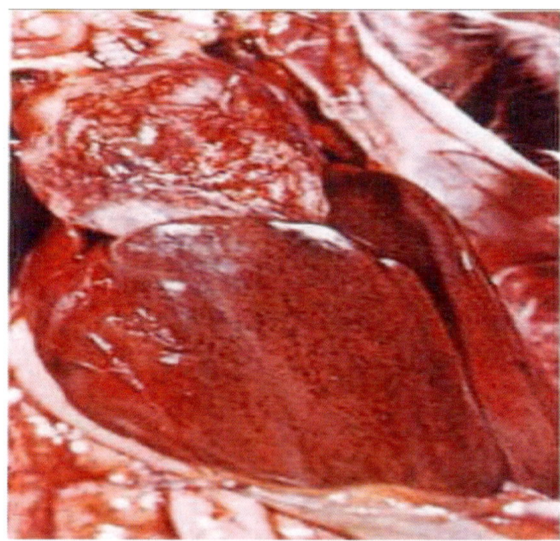

Fig. 15: *E. Coli* infection-enlarged mottled liver and pericarditis.

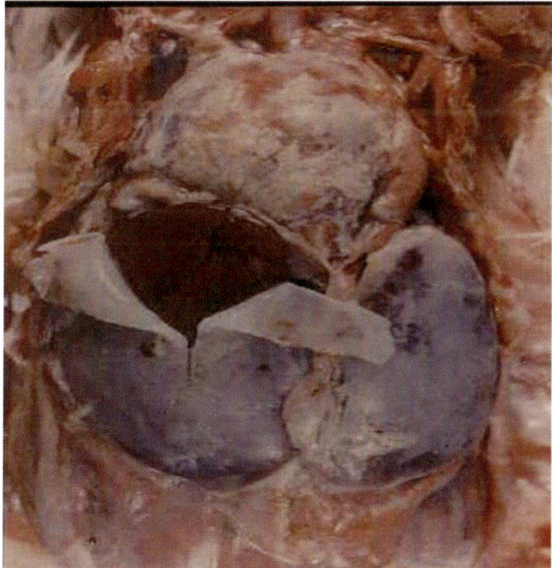

Fig. 16: *E. coli*/mycoplasma complicated case. Severe pericarditis and perihepatitis.

4. Coli granuloma (Hjarre's disease)

Lesions of granuloma may develop in isolated cases in liver, ceca, duodenum and mesentery. The granuloma resembles to lesions of tuberculosis but the staining of sections for acid fast bacteria can help in differentiation of the two conditions. Coli granuloma is not a common condition.

5. Pericarditis

Pericarditis is produced following septicemia. Lesions start as serous but progress quickly to fibrinous inflammation. Myocarditis is accompanied in majority of cases. Organization of exudate results in chronic passive congestion leading to fibrosis of liver.

6. Swollen Head Syndrome (SHS)

SHS results from acute to subacute cellulitis of subcutaneous tissue in the head. Although, *E.coli* is most frequently associated with SHS, it occurs in association with turkey rhinotracheitis virus (TRT) and in condition with poor ventilation and high level of ammonia as predisposing factors. **SHS has been reported recently in turkeys in North Central USA.**

7. Avian Cellulitis *(Inflammatory process, Infectious process or IP)*

Chronic skin disease affecting the abdomen of broiler chickens. Lesions are in the subcutaneous tissue of the skin between thigh and midline; and consist of caseated exudate. **IP is an important cause of carcass condemnation.**

8. Coli Septicemia of Ducks

Lesions of Coli septicemia similar to those caused by *Riemerella anatipestifer* have been reported in ducks (all ages) associated with *E.coli* infections. Liver and spleen are swollen and varying degree pericarditis, perihepatitis and air saculitis with curd like exudate is noticed.

Diagnosis

1. The epidemiology and lesions are suggestive.
2. For final diagnosis isolation and identification of the organism is essential.

Differential Diagnosis

The following conditions must be differentiated in the diagnosis of *E. coli* infection:

1) **Omphalitis:** Salmonellosis, staphylococcal infection, proteus infection, aerobactor, klebsiella and clostridial infections.

2) **Synovitis / arthritis:** *Mycoplasma synoviae* infection, salmonellosis, staphylococcal infection and viral arthritis.

3) **Acute septicemia:** Pasteurellosis (Fowl cholera), salmonellosis and streptococcal infection.

Treatment

E. coli is sensitive to many drugs, such as antibiotics, nitrofurans and sulfa drugs. However, the isolates of poultry are frequently resistant to one or more drugs. Hence, it is advisable to do the drug sensitivity of the *E. coli* isolate involved in the disease, so that effective drug can be used.

Prevention and Control

1) Good husbandry methods, such as avoiding of overcrowding, providing proper ventilation, cleaning and disinfection of houses and equipment between the two crops of chicks, should be practised to reduce the predisposing factors.

2) Raising mycoplasma free birds can also reduce *E. coli* infection. Exposure to other respiratory viruses should also be avoided.

3) Transmission of *E. coli* through faecal contamination can be reduced by fumigation of hatching eggs.

4) All procedures detailed for prevention and control of paratyphoid are applicable for *E. coli* as well.

9

Fowl Cholera

Disease is worldwide in distribution

Etiology

Pasteurella multocida, a gram negative non spore forming, non motile rods which stain bipolar.

Epizootiology

Most species of birds are infected. Turkeys are more susceptible than chickens, and older chickens are more vulnerable than young chickens. Geese and ducks of all ages are highly susceptible to fowl cholera. Survivors of fowl cholera outbreaks become carriers and are the reservoir of infection. ***P. multocida*** **isolates of pigs are pathogenic to fowls**. Spread of *P. multocida* in a flock is by feed and water contaminated with excretions. Crates, feed bags and utensils serve as a mechanical carrier of the organism.

Clinical Signs

1) With acute fowl cholera, the birds may die within 26-48 hours after exposure. There may not be any clinical sign.

2) In subacute cases, main clinical signs are anorexia, drowsiness, fever, diarrhoea, cyanosis and watery discharge from the mouth.

3) Chronic fowl cholera may follow an acute stage of the disease, or it may result from infection with organisms of low virulence. The clinical signs of chronic fowl cholera are related to localisation of disease. The death rate is low, but deaths continue for many months. The infection usually localises in wattles, sinuses, leg/wing joints, foot pad and sternum.

Gross Lesions

Acute and Subacute form

1) The postmortem lesions are associated with vascular disturbances. Wide spread petechial and ecchymotic haemorrhages are found. Sub epicardial and sub serosal haemorrhages are most common. Hemorrhages are also found in lung, abdominal fat and intestinal mucosa.
2) The liver is enlarged, congested and friable with necrotic foci (Figure 17).
3) Ovarian follicles may be flaccid or ruptured.
4) Pneumonia is observed, but more commonly in turkeys. Usually, there is unilateral consolidation of lungs, with fibrinous pleuritis (Figure 18).

Chronic Form

Fluid or caseous exudate may be seen in affected joints, wattles, conjunctival sac, middle ear, and tendon sheath and infraorbital sinuses.

Diagnosis

From clinical history and lesions, a tentative diagnosis may be made. Final diagnosis should be based on isolation and identification of the organism. A tentative diagnosis in acute and subacute cholera can be made by staining the liver impression smears with Giemsa for demonstration of bipolar organisms.

Treatment

Antibiotics and sulfonamides have been used to control the outbreaks. However, drug sensitivity test is of advantage before starting treatment since strains of *P. multocida* vary in susceptibility to chemotherapeutic agents.

Prevention and Control

Since fowl cholera is not a disease of the hatchery, good management practices with emphasis on sanitation are the best way of prevention.

Vaccination

In areas where fowl cholera is endemic, vaccination should be done at 6-8 weeks of age. Second vaccination is given 2 months later. Vaccine is a killed bacterial culture. Immunity lasts for 6-8 months.

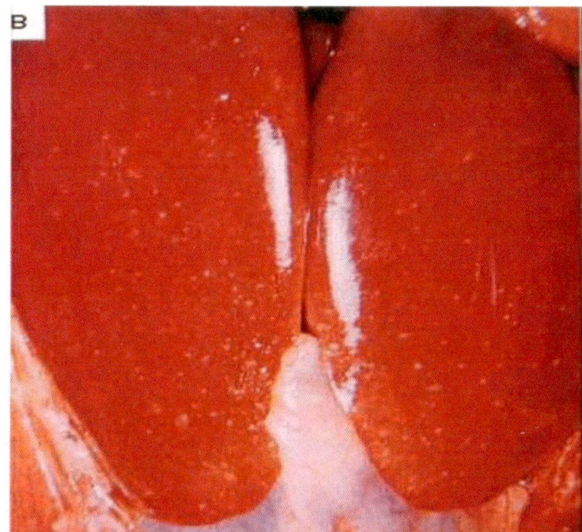

Fig. 17: Liver from a turkey showing enlargement, congestion and multiple white necrotic foci in acute fowl cholera.

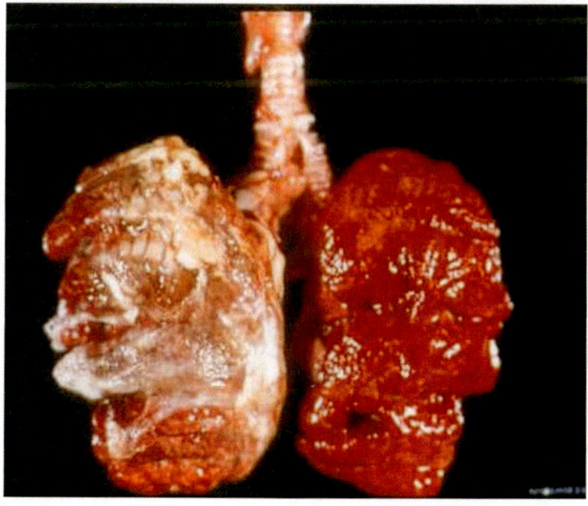

Fig. 18: Unilateral fibrinous pleuritis and pneumonia in turkey in acute fowl cholera.

SECTION-1
Basics About Avian

10

Riemerella Anatipestifer Infection

(New duck disease, Duck septicemia, Anatipestifer syndrome, Infectious Serositis, the disease in goose is called "goose influenza")

Etiology

The disease was first described in ducks from 3 farms in Long Island, N.Y. in 1932. *R. anatipestifer (Pasteurella anatipestifer)* is a gram negative, non-motile, non-spore-forming rod occurring singly, in pairs and occasionally in chains. To date, 19 serotypes are reported.

Natural and experimental hosts: primarily a disease of domestic ducks. Outbreaks also reported in turkeys. Bacteria have been isolated from pheasants, chickens, guinea fowl, quail, partridge and other waterfowl.

Transmission

The organism usually enters the body through the respiratory tract and puncture of the skin. Adverse environmental conditions or concomitant diseases are predisposing factors for the outbreaks.

Clinical Signs

Disease in ducklings between 1 and eight weeks is severe with mortality varying from 5 to 75%. Mild coughing, sneezing, ocular and nasal discharge are initial signs. Final stages show greenish diarrhoea. A few may develop nervous signs, which include ataxia, tremor of the head and neck and birds may go into the coma.

Lesions

The most significant gross lesion is fibrinous exudate on serosal surfaces in general but is most evident on the pericardium and the liver. Also, fibrinous air saculitis involving thoracic and abdominal air sacs, caseous salpingitis and arthritis are also observed. The lesions in CNS consist of fibrinous meningitis. Chronically infected ducks have necrotic dermatitis.

Diagnosis and Differential Diagnosis

Many septicemic infections like *Streptococci, Escherichia coli, and Chlamydia* produce similar lesions. Hence isolation and identification of the organism confirms the diagnosis.

Treatment, Prevention and Control

These are similar to those described for fowl cholera. Inactivated bacterins containing serotype 1, 2, and 5 given at 2 and 3 weeks of age provide excellent protection up to the market age of ducks. Oil- emulsion bacterin has been reported to provide better protection. A live vaccine administered aerosol or in drinking water at one day age has been reported to provide significant protection.

11

Erysipelas

Etiology

Erysipelothrix rhusiopathiae.

Disease Occurrence

The disease is worldwide in distribution.

Host Range

Outbreaks of significant economic loss are in turkeys. Occasional outbreaks have been reported in pheasants, ducks, geese, guinea fowl, chukars, grebes and emus. Erysipelas also occurs in swine, sheep, sea mammals, fish and many wild animals. In humans (fish handlers, butchers, kitchen workers, turkey growers and veterinarians) it causes a localised inflammation called "erysipeloid".

Transmission

The actual mode of transmission is not well established. However, following two routes are speculated. Organisms are shed in faeces of infected birds, sheep and swine and contaminate the soil, water and feed. The oral route is believed to be the route of natural infection. Organisms can enter the body through breaks in the skin or mucous membranes. Male turkeys are considered to get the infection through this route, via wounds caused in the fight. Females are reported infected during AI through infected semen.

Clinical Signs

The onset of disease in turkey flocks is sudden, with a few birds found dead. These deaths are usually suspected of poisoning, stampede or predators. Careful examination of flock reveals a few sleepy depressed birds. Most sick birds die suddenly, probably as a result of emboli. Male turkeys show swollen snood. Dark bruised lesions are found on face and head.

Chronically affected birds show gradual emaciation, anaemia and death. These are birds having lesions of endocarditis.

Lesions

Lesions are those of generalised septicemia. Hemorrhages are marked on abdominal fat, heart muscles, thigh muscles and serous membranes. Liver, spleen, kidneys are swollen and mottled. There is a varying degree of skin reddening, especially on face, neck and head. Other lesions include fibrinopurulent exudate in joints. Vegetative valvular endocarditis is seen in a few dead birds. Sudden losses in hens following AI are marked with lesions of peritonitis.

Diagnosis

1. History, clinical signs and septicemic lesions may give a presumptive diagnosis. Isolation and identification (which is not easy and constant) should provide confirmation.
2. Gram stained smears from the tissues will reveal Gram positive slightly curved thin bacilli. FAT on smears or tissue sections is useful.
3. Differential diagnosis: a) from fowl cholera- Splenomegaly in erysipelas and pneumonia in fowl cholera. b) from other acute septicemia- *E. coli, Salmonella, Chlamydia* and *Streptococci.*

Treatment

A rapid acting form of penicillin should be used on sick birds. Sodium or potassium salts of penicillin at a rate of 10,000U/lb. body wt. is administered IM. Simultaneous injection of erysipelas bacterin is advantageous. The combination of water-soluble penicillin and long acting penicillin to the whole flock is beneficial, if cost effective.

Prevention and Control

General bio-security measures.

Vaccination

Formalin- inactivated, aluminium hydroxide adsorbed the whole cell *E. rhusiopathiae* bacterins are widely used. Vaccinate turkeys at 8-12 wk old by S/C route at the dorsal surface of the neck behind the atlas. Breeder turkeys are vaccinated twice at a 4-wk interval before the onset of egg production. Recently, use of a live vaccine in experimental groups has been reported with better efficacy.

12

Yersinia Pseudotuberculosis (Pasteurella Pseudotuberculosis)

Etiology

Yersinia pseudotuberculosis, non-motile at 37 °C but motile at room temperature around 25 C. It is a disease of turkeys, ducks, geese, chickens, guinea fowl, and companion birds and free flying birds. It has also been reported in many species of mammals including man. In man, it causes symptoms of appendicitis. The disease has been reported in many countries. Body excretions of diseased birds or mammals that contaminate soil, food and water are the important factor in the transmission of the disease. The disease usually occurs as an acute septicemia of short duration, followed by a chronic focal infection.

Clinical Signs

Vary considerably

1. In very acute cases, birds may die suddenly without symptoms; where disease extends over two weeks or more, birds show weakness, ruffled feathers, difficulty in breathing, diarrhoea, emaciation and paralysis. In acute cases, swelling of the spleen and enteritis are main lesions. In chronic cases, liver and spleen are enlarged. Yellowish white necrotic foci resembling lesions of tuberculosis may be found in the liver, lung, spleen and breast muscles. There is usually severe hemorrhagic enteritis.
2. *Yersinia pseudotuberculosis* causes a granulomatous lesion in the liver of psittacines.
3. No useful treatment or vaccine is available.
4. Sanitary and hygienic measures are followed for prevention and control.

13

Campylobacter Infections

Etiology

There are 18 species in genus Campylobacter. Campylobacter species in poultry include *C. jejuni, C. coli* and *C. lari.* The most predominant species is *C. jejuni.*

Epizootiology

The infection has been reported in chicken, but the organisms have been isolated from ducks, turkeys, black birds, sparrow and pigeons.

Transmission

Possibly through faeces, as organisms are in the intestinal tract. Egg transmission of bacteria on or in the egg through hatchery is strongly suggested.

In broilers

No apparent gross pathology or clinical disease has been reported. Campylobacter organisms are found on the chicken carcass at slaughter. Isolation studies have shown that 75% of live broilers and 80% of poultry meat are contaminated. Organisms survive carcass-processing operations at slaughter. *Campylobacter* from poultry are being shown as primary sources of gastroenteritis in man; hence an emerging zoonotic problem. Handling and consumption of contaminated poultry or poultry products induce disease in humans.

In layers

The organism has been associated with hepatitis in pullets, coming in production. Clinical outbreaks usually follow stress caused by other diseases, like worm infestation, Marek's disease, Fowl pox, E. coli, mycoplasma and coccidiosis.

Clinical Signs

1) The disease runs a chronic course. The affected flock fails to reach a peak production.
2) The individual birds show loss of weight, anaemia and gradual emaciation.
3) There is diarrhoea in the affected flock. Mortality is low ranging between 2 to 5%.

Gross Lesions

1) The lesions are mainly in the liver, but are variable and not observed in all clinically positive birds. Initial liver lesions consist of enlargement of the organ and the presence of small irregular necrotic foci. Areas of haemorrhages and sometimes rupture of the liver are also found. The severely affected liver has a large cauliflower like necrotic areas throughout the liver.
2) Chronic cases show cirrhosis of the liver accompanied with ascites and hydropericardium.
3) The spleen is enlarged and necrotic. The heart may also show necrosis.

Diagnosis

History of the flock and gross lesions are suggestive. For confirmation, isolation and identification of the organism are necessary. However, isolation of the organisms is not always successful. Liver, spleen, kidneys, bile, heart, pericardial fluid and intestinal contents are specimens for culture. Isolation can be done in:

1. Artificial media
2. Developing chicken embryos

ELISA, FAT, and PCR based methods are currently in use for quick and accurate diagnosis.

Differential Diagnosis

Need to be differentiated from other diseases, which have lesions in the liver, like pullorum diseases, fowl typhoid, fowl cholera, leukosis, tuberculosis, quails disease.

Treatment and Control

Treatment with furazolidone, tetracyclines and injectable streptomycin has given good results, but relapses have been observed even after treatment.

Vaccination

No vaccine is available. Hygienic measures are recommended for prevention and control of Campylobacter infection.

14

Spirochetosis

Causative Organism: *Borrelia anserina*

B. anserina and *B. burgdorferi* (borreliosis of humans) share common flagellar antigens, suggesting their close relationship. *B. burgdorferi* infect both mammals and birds (mallards and bobwhite quail). Geese, turkeys, chickens, ducks, pheasants and canaries are natural hosts of *B. anserina.* All age birds are susceptible.

Transmission

Infection is mainly transmitted by a soft tick- *Argus persicus.* Transmission is also by ingestion of blood, excreta or tissues from infected or dead birds, through contaminated feed or water. Use of syringe and needles on multiple birds also makes transmission possible.

Clinical Signs

Usually, after 3-8 days of incubation, there is a high rise of body temperature, accompanied by the appearance of the organism in the blood. In chronic stages of the disease, the organisms disappear from the blood, also from the tissues. There are no specific clinical signs. However, infected birds become anaemic, depressed with ruffled feathers. They may develop greenish diarrhoea and finally may become paralytic. Morbidity varies from 10 to 100%. Similarly, mortality is also variable from 2-to100%, depending on the pathogenicity of the strain.

Gross Lesions

There is marked enlargement of spleen with ecchymotic haemorrhages. The liver may be enlarged, congested and contain small areas of necrosis. Kidneys are pale and show nephrotic changes.

Diagnosis

The demonstration of spirochetes in stained blood smears or wet preparations by dark field microscope. Spirochetes may not be found during the last phase of the disease. Isolation of organisms in embryonated chicken or turkey eggs. The use of agar gel precipitation test and FAT in the diagnosis has been reported.

Treatment

Antibiotics especially penicillin, streptomycin, amphomycin, tetracycline and chloromycetin have been useful in the treatment.

Prevention and Control

Control of ticks and mosquitoes is important in prevention. Recovered and vaccinated birds are immune for an extended period.

Vaccination

Many types of bacterins have been useful. Usually given IM at 6-8 weeks of age. Immunity is type specific; hence multi-serotype or autogenous vaccines are necessary.

15

Avian Intestinal Spirochetosis

Etiology

Intestinal spirochetes colonise the large intestine of avian, swine and humans.

Family spirochaetacae has six genera, of which Borrelia, Serpulina and Treponema have species pathogenic for animals. Avian intestinal spirochetes are grouped in four: *Serpulina hyodysenteriae, S. intermedius, S. pilosicoli (Angullina coli)* and an unnamed group.

Chicken *S. hyodysenteriae* is different from porcine one. *S. hyodysentriae, Angullina coli* and unclassified groups are present in the USA, whereas *S.intermedius* is in Europe and Australia.

Avian intestinal spirochetes are gram negative, stain brown with silver impregnation techniques and blue in Wright-Giemsa stain. They can be divided in 3 pathotypes 1) severely pathogenic 2) Mildly to moderate pathogenic and 3) subclinical or apathogenic.

Host Range

They infect chickens, common rheas, grouse, pheasants, turkeys and wild birds. Naturally, an occurring disease is in rheas.

Transmission is by the fecal-oral route.

Clinical Signs and Lesions

S. hyodysenteriae produces severe disease in rheas, while S. intermedius produces moderate and *A. coli* and unclassified groups produce average to apathogenic disease in chickens and wild ducks.

Disease in rheas produces necrotic typhlitis with a mortality rate ranging from 25 to 80%. The disease is more common in young adult rheas more than six months old. Infected rheas pass watery faeces and die suddenly without clinical signs. Ceca is dilated and show ulceration.

Diagnosis

1. Demonstration of bacteria in faecal samples by dark field microscopy.
2. The demonstration of spirochete antigen.
3. The culture of spirochetes.
4. Serology: Agar gel diffusion test (AGDT) has been used in birds. Other serological methods like ELISA, indirect FAT, passive hemolysis assay and micro-agglutination test used for swine could be applied to birds.

Differential Diagnosis

The presence of spirochetes in faecal samples is differentiated from other spiral bacteria like Campylobacter, Arcobacter, Helicobacter and Spirillum. In rheas, other bacteria like *Salmonella, Clostridium spp*. (*C. perfringens, C.sordelli and C.difficile*) and *Histomonas meleagridis* cause necrotizing typhlitis. Lesions in ceca caused by eastern equine encephalomyelitis virus (EEEV) also resemble spirochete infection. However, EEEV produces widespread lesions of necrosis and haemorrhages in the small intestine and other organs.

Treatment

5- nitroimidazole in water (120 ppm) for six days is effective in birds. Repeat treatment after 4-8 weeks may be required. For rheas, dimetridozole (25-50 mg/kg-body wt., once or twice daily), lincomycin (25 mg/kg twice daily) or erythromycin (15-25 mg/kg-body wt.) for 5-7 days has been used with success.

Prevention and Control

It is a severe disease in rheas. Hence strict biosecurity measures should be implemented to minimise its introduction in rheas. No vaccine is available.

16

Clostridial Infections

In avian species following diseases are caused by Clostridium bacteria.

1. Ulcerative enteritis
2. Necrotic enteritis
3. Gangrenous Dermatitis
4. Botulism
5. Yolk sac infections.

Clostridia infections are not common in birds and are not a significant source of infection for man and animals.

ULCERATIVE ENTERITIS

(Quail Disease)

The disease is world wide in distribution.

Causative Bacteria

A new species of clostridia- C. colinum.

Epizootiology

Ulcerative enteritis is found in most avian species, but quail are most susceptible. The disease is also reported in toucans and ratites.

Clinical Signs and Lesions

Birds dying in the acute stage show no clinical signs. In sub acute phase birds are depressed with ruffled feathers. Chronic stages show atrophy of muscles and extreme emaciation. In chickens mortality range from 2 to 10% and recovery is common. Quail have 100% mortality. The gross lesions are in the intestines followed by liver and the spleen. Intestine and ceca show ulcers and necrosis. Initially, the ulcers are small, superficial and circular with hemorrhagic borders.

Ulcers increase in size and small ulcers join to form big necrotic diphtheritic patches. Perforations of ulcers commonly occur resulting in peritonitis and intestinal adhesions. The necrotic lesions in the liver are pale yellow or grey and are a pinhead to several centimetres in size. The spleen is enlarged, congested and sometimes hemorrhagic.

Diagnosis

1. Gross lesions in the intestine and liver are suggestive for clinical diagnosis.
2. Confirmation is done by crushing a necrotic piece of liver between two slides, fixed by heat and stained with Gram stain. Large Gram positive rods with spores confirms the diagnosis.
3. Complement fixation and FAT are rapid methods of diagnosis.
4. Differential Diagnosis: From the diseases that cause similar lesions; Coccidiosis, Histomoniasis, Necrotic enteritis (no infectivity to quail), Hemorrhagic syndrome and Inclusion body hepatitis.

Treatment, Prevention and Control

Antibiotics such as streptomycin in drinking water, chloromycetin and bacitracin in feed have been found useful. Strict biosecurity measures.

NECROTIC ENTERITIS

Causative Organism: *Clostridium perfringens, type A or C*

Epizootiology

Outbreaks of necrotic enteritis occur only sporadically in broiler chicken between 4 and eight weeks of age. Necrotic enteritis also reported in ostrich and psittacines.

Clinical Signs and Lesions

The clinical signs resemble those of coccidiosis. Mortality range between 5 and 50%. Main lesions are in the distal third of the intestine. The wall is congested and thickened. The lumen contains foul smelling brown fluid material. Extensive velvet like necrosis of epithelium is seen. The liver is congested and may contain numerous 2-3 cm diameter necrotic foci.

Diagnosis

Careful microscopic examination of smears and scrapings of the affected part of the intestine is essential to differentiate necrotic enteritis from coccidiosis. In dual infection with coccidiosis (*E. brunetti and E. maxima* which produce similar lesions) culture for clostridia may help in diagnosis.

Treatment and Prevention

Antibiotics such as streptomycin, penicillin and bacitracin are useful in treatment and prophylaxis. Biosecurity is helpful in prevention.

GANGRENOUS DERMATITIS

Etiology

The exact cause of gangrenous dermatitis is still not well known. At least two organisms are implicated. *C. perfringens type A and C. septicum*, but in many outbreaks *S. aureus* and *E. coli* are also involved. Since *clostridia* and *Staphylococci* are the common inhabitants of skin, infection usually follows wounds and injuries that cause initial necrosis, necessary for the growth of clostridia. The staphylococci help to produce anaerobic condition for clostridia growth. The disease occurs in 4-16 weeks old chickens and turkeys. Mortality does not exceed more than 5%.

Clinical Signs and Lesions

There is necrosis of skin and deeper tissues of thighs, breast, lumber region, wing tips, wattles and feet.Underlying muscles show hemorrhagic necrosis with gas. The liver is usually swollen, greenish and may have necrotic areas. Kidney and other visceral organs may show petechial haemorrhages and septicemic changes.

Treatment and Control

Drinking water treatment with streptomycin, penicillin or bacitracin is useful. The prevention of injuries and wounds would reduce the incidence of gangrenous dermatitis.

CLOSTRIDIUM DIFFICILE

Causes enterotyphlocolitis in ratites (Ostrich). Lesions are in the liver in the form of necrotic foci.

BOTULISM

(Limber Neck, Western duck sickness)

Etiology

Botulism is a toxaemia caused by a toxin produced by *C. botulinum*. Botulism neurotoxin is most toxic substance. At least six types of *C. botulinum* are known. The recorded outbreaks in birds have been due to type C. sometimes type B and E are also reported in birds. The causes of human botulism are type A, B and E.

Epizootiology

The organism itself does not produce disease, but its presence in the intestine causes its rapid multiplication in a dead and putrefying carcass. The toxin is produced in such carcass. Botulism occurs by eating toxin-containing carcass. Maggots and fly larvae feeding on such carcass become toxic. High level of toxin is also produced in mud, decaying vegetation and anaerobic organic matter such as feed. Sometimes in broilers *C. botulinum* produces toxin in the intestine, which get absorbed in the body, producing outbreak of botulism (toxico-infectious botulism). Most species of birds are susceptible to botulism, but severe outbreaks have been among the waterfowls.

Clinical Signs and Lesions

Birds become sick within a few hours to 1 or 2 days after ingestion of toxic material. There is weakness and in the coordination of the legs and wings due to paralysis of muscles. Mostly noticed in the neck muscles, causing characteristic **"limber neck",** a name sometimes used for the disease (Figure 19). Birds usually die in coma, from respiratory failure. If a small dose of toxin is ingested, recovery takes place after mild signs of in coordination. There are no gross or microscopic lesions.

Diagnosis

Characteristic paralytic signs in the absence of gross lesions suggest botulism. Diagnosis can be confirmed by the demonstration of toxin, by injecting serum or extract of intestinal content from sick bird, intraperitoneally (0.3ml) into mice. Positive cases develop paralysis in 1-2 days.

Treatment

Administration of *C. botulinum* type C antitoxin controls mortality. Antibiotics with vitamin supplement are useful in toxico infectious botulism.

Prevention

Good management and hygiene normally prevent outbreaks of botulism.

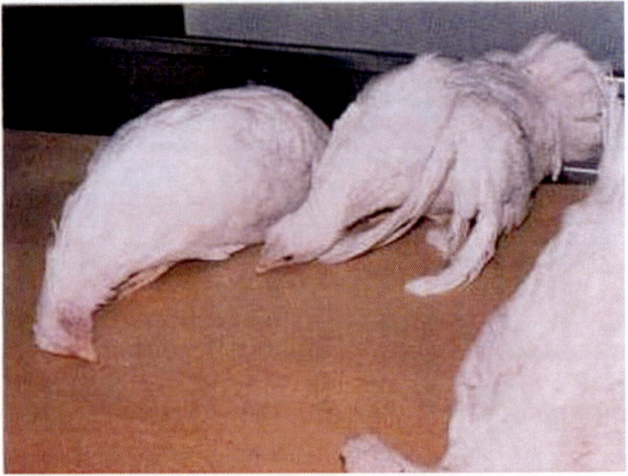

Fig.19: *Clostridium botulinum* infection. Birds showing "limberneck" characteristic of Botulism.

17

Infectious Coryza (Fowl Coryza)

Etiology

Avibacter paragallinarum Serotype A, B *and* C. *Based on hemagglutinin serotyping, three serotypes (A, B and C) have been recognized.*

Epizootiology

The chicken is the natural host although the disease has occasionally been diagnosed in pheasants. All ages of chicken are susceptible but birds up to 10 weeks are less vulnerable.

1) The chronic or healthy carrier birds serve as source of infection. Infection within farm occurs by contact with drinking water or feed contaminated by nasal discharge from sick/carrier chickens. To farms situated at a distance, infection is through air borne transmission.

2) The disease occurs more in cold and wet conditions. The more severe disease occurs when other respiratory diseases are prevalent at the farm.

Clinical Signs and Gross Lesions

1. Rapid spread, high morbidity and low mortality characterize the disease.
2. Clinical signs develop within a week after the infection, which includes serous or mucoid nasal discharge, conjunctivitis and oedema of the face.
3. In advanced cases where the disease has spread to trachea and air sacs, the respiratory rales are heard.
4. A foul odour is present in the flocks, particularly when disease runs a chronic course.
5. Gross lesions include inflammation of nasal passages and sinuses and subcutaneous oedema of the face, wattles and around the eyes. Swelling of infra-orbital sinuses which cause closing of the eyes (Figure 20). Pus develops in the infraorbital sinuses.

Diagnosis

1. A history of rapidly developing respiratory disease with coryza like clinical signs is suggestive of the diagnosis. For confirmation, isolation and identification of the organism are essential. Best specimen for culture is swab taken from the infraorbital sinus where organism is usually found in pure culture. Tracheal and air sac swabs can also be used for culture.
2. Tube agglutination, hemagglutination inhibition and fluorescent antibody tests, ELISA and PCR based molecular techniques are useful in diagnosis.
3. Confirmation could be made by inoculation of susceptible chicken into the sinuses with exudate or culture suspension. Coryza like clinical signs appears in 24-48 hours.
4. Differential diagnosis: infectious coryza must be differentiated from CRD, chronic fowl cholera, fowl pox and Vitamin A deficiency which produce similar lesions.

Treatment

Sulfonamide and antibiotics are useful in checking the severity of the disease. No drug has been found bactericidal; hence, outbreaks recur after the treatment is discontinued and birds remain carriers.

Prevention and Control

Since recovered carrier birds are the main source of infection, starter birds should not be purchased from the infected flock. Once the outbreak has occurred in a flock, it is advisable to depopulate the flock.

Vaccine

In some countries, the vaccine made up of formalin killed culture with adjuvant is available. Two doses of vaccine are given subcutaneously at a four weeks interval. The first vaccination is given at about 10-12 weeks of age. Immunity lasts for at least seven months. The dose is 0.5 ml subcutaneously preferably in the breast region.

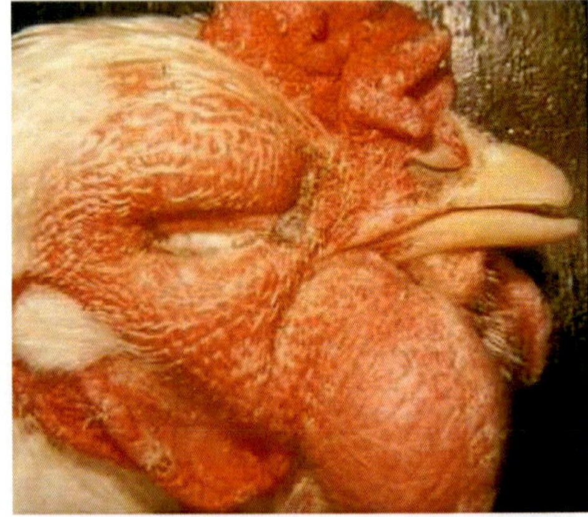

Fig. 20: Infectious coryza; edema of face, wattles and around the eyes causing closing of the eye

18

Ornithobacterium Rhinotracheale Infection

Etiology

Ornithobacteriun rhinotracheale, bacteria, under phylum Cytophaga-Flavobacterium-Bacteroids. It is Gram negative non-motile, non-sporulating pleomorphic rod shaped bacteria. 18 serotypes A through R have been identified. Serotype A is prevalent in chicken and turkeys.

Disease occurrence

The disease is worldwide in distribution.

Hosts

O. rhinotracheale has been isolated from many species of birds including chicken and turkey. In commercial poultry, the disease is more common in older birds.

Transmission

O. rhinotracheale spreads horizontally through aerosols and contaminated drinking water. Vertical transmission is indicated.

Clinical Signs

1) Clinical signs are observed within 24 hours post infection.
2) In younger (3-6 week old) broilers main symptoms are nasal discharge, sneezing, facial swelling, decreased feed intake with a mortality rate of 2% to 10%.
3) In breeders, mild respiratory signs with the reduction in feed intake are primary symptoms. There is drop in egg production with small size and poor egg shell quality.
4) Similar clinical signs are also observed in turkey.

Pathology

Gross lesions: include pneumonia, airsacculitis and pleuritis. Pneumonia is either unilateral or bilateral with fibrinous pleuritis. Microscopically there are fibrinous inflammatory lesions in lungs, along with necrotic foci.

Diagnosis

Clinical signs are diagnostic, but confirmatory diagnosis is base on isolation and identification of bacterium. Trachea, lungs and air sacs are the best tissue for isolation. Bacterial media are used for culture. PCR based method is preferred for quick diagnosis. Other methods employed are FAT and ELIZA.

Differential Diagnosis

Because of similarity of clinical signs produced by *E. coli, Avibacterium paragallinarum, R. anatipestfer and Chlamydophila psittaci* a critical diagnostic evaluation be made.

Treatment, Prevention and Control

Because of variability in susceptibility of strains *O. rhinotracheale* with various antibiotics, treatment is difficult. Strict biosecurity measures are applied to prevent the introduction of the disease on the farm premises.Vaccination of breeders is advisable to protect the progeny. Commercial vaccines are available.

19

Bardetellosis (Turkey Coryza)

An important disease in Turkey producing areas of the world. It is reported an opportunistic pathogen to human. Bactria grows in ciliated epithelium of vertebrates.

Etiology

Bordetella avium, a small Gram-negative bacillus, which is motile and aerobic. Differences in pathogenicity among strains exist.

Transmission

Recovered birds serve as carriers. Turkey coryza is highly contagious, and transmission occurs directly through close contact and contaminated feed and water.

Clinical Signs

1) The incubation period is short (7-10 days).
2) The natural disease occurs in young (2-6 week old) poults.
3) Lesions are confined to the upper respiratory tract and vary with the time.
4) Initial lesions include catarrhal nasal discharge, frothy ocular discharge, sneezing, snicking and flicking of head. Later exudate becomes crusted brown and seen sticking to head nares and feathers.
5) Infra orbital sinuses may be swollen.
6) Many poults show mouth breathing and dyspnea.
7) Morbidity is very high (80%), but mortality is low (10%).

Lesions

1) Mucus to mucopurulent tracheitis as the disease progress.

2) Distortion of tracheal cartilage because of softening and weakness of chondrocytes. In isolated cases, there is dorsal- ventral in folding of tracheal wall into the lumen, more prominent immediately below the larynx. Fibrinopurulent exudate is found in the tracheal lumen.

Diagnosis

Clinical signs of the disease are indicative of tentative diagnosis. Isolation and identification of bacteria may confirm the diagnosis. *B. avium* is HA positive with guinea pig blood. Pathogenicity test may be performed by intranasal inoculation of day-old poults. For serological test ELISA, and FAT are useful.

Differential Diagnosis

Bardetellosis must be differentiated from Mycoplasmosis, Chlamydiosis which produce rhinotracheitis.

20

Mycobacteriosis

Etiology

Genus Mycobacterium contains many pathogenic species that can cause disease in birds (*M. avium, M. tuberculosis, M. genavenes, M. gordonae).* Within *M. avium,* organisms are divided into four sub species. *M. avium sp avium, M.avium sp silvaticum, M. avium sp homnissuis* and *M. avium sp paratuberculosis. Mycobacterium avium sp avium* - has wide host spectrum; poultry, pigeons, raptors, ratites and wild birds. M. *genavense*- affects Psittacines and passarines. *M. tuberculosis*- psittacines and other cage birds, and wild birds in captivity. *M.bovis*- Psittacines and others.

Under natural conditions, *M. avium sp avium* does not cause severe disease in mammals except in rabbit and pig. Majority of mycobacteriosis in pigs is by *M. avium sp avium.* In cattle and other mammal infection by *M. avium* remain localized and is known to give positive reaction to mammalian tuberculin. The disease in caged and wild birds in captivity is common with *M. tuberculosis*, because of its close contact with humans. Tuberculosis is a serious problem in zoological gardens. *M. avium* is being isolated in increasing number of immunocompromized human patients.

Distribution

Tuberculosis in chickens is world wide in distribution.

Transmission

The ulcerative lesions of tuberculosis in the intestine of poultry are the primary source of bacteria in faeces. Bacteria are also discharged in faeces if lesions are in liver and gall bladder. Lesions in trachea contaminate environment through droplet infection. Premises also get infected from infected swine and wild birds. Bacteria are quite resistant. Hence premises remain infected for longer period and remain a source of infection.

Clinical Signs

Birds of all ages are susceptible, but symptoms and lesions are more in older birds because the disease progresses slowly. The affected birds show progressive loss of weight, with atrophy of pectoral and breast muscles. The breastbone becomes prominent giving a "knife edged" appearance. The anaemic changes are seen in comb, wattles and ear lobes. The skin over shank is dry. If lesions are in bone marrow, the bird will show unilateral or bilateral paralysis with jerky movement. Most affected chickens have lesions in the intestine resulting in chronic diarrhoea.

Lesions

1) Lesions are most consistently seen in liver, spleen, intestine and bone marrow.
2) Lesions are in the form of irregular greyish yellow or greyish white nodules varying from pin- head to several centimetres in diameter (Figure 21). The surface of the nodules is uneven with small granulations. Cut surface of the nodules may contain small yellow caseous foci. Nodules can be easily enucleated.
3) The nodules in the intestine usually involve the whole thickness of the intestine. The majority of nodules have ulcerated surface on the mucosal surface.

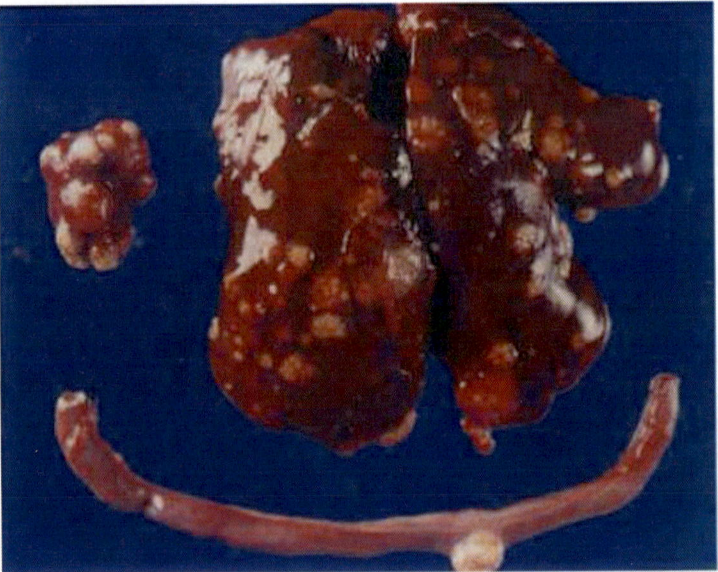

Fig. 21: Mycobacteriosis (yellowish caseous nodules in liver, intestine and spleen)

Diagnosis

1. The demonstration of acid fast bacilli in smears and tissue sections.
2. Pathogenicity test: into chickens or rabbit. The guinea pig is refractory to *M. avium*.
3. Tuberculin test: It is a flock test.
4. Whole blood agglutination test
5. Culture of organism
6. ELISA test
7. PCR based method

Differential Diagnosis

1) Bacteria producing necrotic lesions in liver and spleen- Salmonella, Pasteurella, Campylobacter and chlamydia. (The absence of acid fast bacilli in impression smears.)
2) The fungi with granuloma. (Characteristic fungal hyphae.)
3) Histomoniasis in liver.
4) Neoplasms in liver and spleen. (Cut surfaces of a tumour are uniform without necrosis.)

Treatment

The treatment is uneconomical.

Prevention and Control

1) Reactors are detected by tuberculin test or blood test. It is better to depopulate the positive flock because even a single bird will contaminate the premises again.
2) Swine and chicken should not be kept together.

21

Chlamydiosis

Chlamydial organisms are spherical 0.2-1.5 um in diameter. They can be stained and seen in the light microscope, but they grow only in living cells. Chlamydial organisms infect mammals and birds causing various disease syndromes. Chlamydiacae family has one genus; Chlamydia. *C. trachomatis, C. suis* and *C. muridarum.* They cause disease in man, swine and mice. *C. psittaci, C. pneumonia, C. felis, C. Caviae*, and *C. abortus.* cause disease in man, birds and animals. Species can be differentiated on their growth characters inside the host cell.

AVIAN CHLAMYDIOSIS (AC)

(Psittacosis – in humans and psittacine birds; Ornithosis – in any bird other than a psittacine)

AC is caused by *C. psittaci. C. psittaci* has six serotypes named A to F. It affects domestic as well as wild birds. The disease is of economic importance in pigeons, turkey and ducks and less frequently in chickens and geese. Wild birds act as reservoirs. The disease is of public health importance.

Depending on the pathogenicity, strains of *C. psittaci* have been grouped into two Classes:

1) Virulent strains (toxigenic strains)

Isolated most often from turkeys. They cause high mortality, sometimes up to 30%. They are highly pathogenic to mice and other laboratory hosts. This strain causes infection in man; usually in research workers and poultry handlers.

2) Low virulent strains

Causes slow disease with less than 5% mortality. This type is mostly isolated from pigeons and ducks.

Transmission

Large numbers of chlamydia organisms are excreted in faeces of infected birds. In pigeons, organisms are also excreted in nasal discharge. In turkey, when organisms are localized in nasal glands, they are excreted in nasal discharge. Organisms remain infectious for many months in dried excrements. Infection to new host is through inhalation of infected excreta/ dust.

In wild carriers and cage birds, a delicate host-parasite relationship is established, and under stress, these carriers intermittently shed organisms in their secretions and excretions.

A few cage birds (Finches, Canaries and Mynahs) have highly fatal disease, hence do not serve as reservoirs of chlamydia.

Clinical Signs and Lesions

The incubation period, morbidity and mortality are variable depending on the age of the host and pathogenicity of the strain. Clinical signs may develop as quick as 5-10 days or delayed for 2-8 weeks. The lesions are mainly in the liver, spleen and serous membranes.

In Turkeys

Turkeys infected with virulent strains show anorexia and high fever. Droppings become gelatinous yellow green. Egg production declines rapidly. Low virulent strains do not affect egg production. Lungs show diffuse congestion and pleural cavity contains fibrinous exudate.

Pericardium shows fibrinous pericarditis. The liver is enlarged, discoloured and coated with fibrin (Figure 22) Necrotic foci may also be present. Spleen is enlarged, dark red in colour. A rare manifestation in turkeys is nasal gland infection by localization of organism in the nasal glands. It causes characteristic swelling on the head. Sero- fibrinous exudate seen in different parts of the body contains a large number of mononuclear cells. Chlamydia organisms are present in the cytoplasm of mononuclear cells.

In Ducks

It is a debilitating often-fatal disease in ducks. Young ducks develop trembling imbalanced gait. They show anorexia and watery green faeces. They produce serous or purulent discharge from the eyes and nostrils causing the feathers on head encrusted. Morbidity is high up to 80%, but mortality varies and may reach 30% in concurrent infections. Lesions are similar to those as in turkeys. In recent years, in some outbreaks, the lesions were minimum or absent.

In Psittacines

During active chlamydiosis, clinical signs include conjunctivitis (Cockatiels) rhinitis, diarrhoea, polyuria, dyspnea, tail-bobbing and icterus (especially in macaw). Less frequently are signs of torticollis and leg paralysis. Some infected birds show wax-and-wane course with period of illness followed by apparent good health. Lesions are similar to those in pigeons.

In Pigeons (parrot fever)

Infection is believed to be transmitted by a parent-to—nestling feeding. In the acute phase, pigeons are anorectic and diarrheic. Some develop conjunctivitis, swollen eyelids and rhinitis. Respiratory difficulty results in rattling sound. Chronically affected pigeons show weakness and die. Some recover and become carriers. Significant amounts of urate are found in faecal content. Chlamydial bodies are reported in renal tubular epithelium. Other lesions are similar to those described for turkeys.

In Chickens

Chickens appear to be relatively resistant. However, in clinical cases, lesions of conjunctivitis, pericarditis, perihepatitis and air saculitis have been reported.

Diagnosis

It is based on isolation and identification of the organisms and demonstration of rising antibody titer in circulation of infected birds.

- **Specimen required:** Fibrinous exudate is the best specimen for isolation. Lung, liver, spleen along with exudate can also be used for isolation. Isolation is done in following host system.
- **Tissue culture:** Human and mice cell cultures are used.
- **Chicken embryos:** Five to seven-day old chicken embryos are inoculated through yolk sac route. Organisms grow in yolk and cause death of embryos in 3-10 days after inoculation. Organisms can be demonstrated in yolk.
- **Mice Inoculation:** Mice can be infected by intra- peritoneal or intranasal route. Ascites and splenomegaly develop in positive cases.
- **Microscopic demonstration of organisms:** *C. psittasi* can be seen in mononuclear cells in wet mount under phase contrast microscope (Figure 23). The organisms are also seen after staining in smears prepared from exudate or impression smears of organs. Chlamydia stain well with Giemsa, Machiavillo or Gimenez stains. Smears can also be examined stained with fluorescin conjugated specific antibodies.

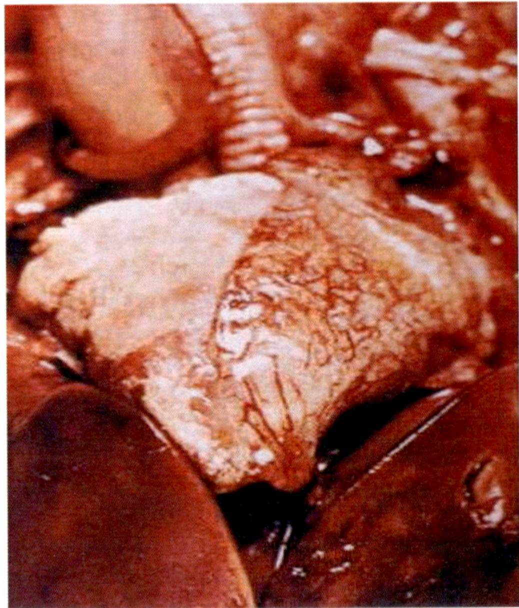

Fig. 22: Chlamydiosis in a turkey (pericarditis, enlarged liver)

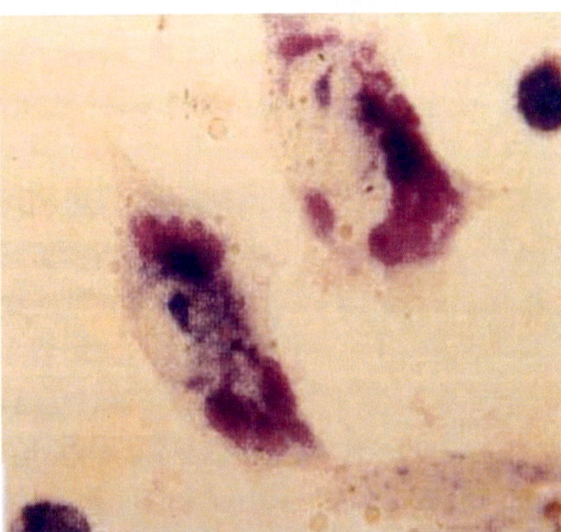

Fig. 23: Chlamydia species stained with Giemsa; organisms seen in mononuclear cells.

Serology

AGPT and micro- complement fixation methods are used to detect antibodies. Four folds or greater increase in serum antibodies in infected birds is considered diagnostic. Recently, ELISA is method of choice. PCR is being used in the diagnosis of human chlamydiosis.

Treatment

Tetracycline given in feed or water for two weeks controls the infection. In pigeons, the treatment is repeated many times after two weeks to remove the infection from carrier birds.

Prevention and Control

There is no commercial vaccine. Prevention of disease should be through strict biosecurity methods. The disease is reportable and must be reported to appropriate authorities. Flocks should be treated and slaughtered under supervision.

22

Omphalitis (Navel ill, Mushy chick disease)

Etiology

Mostly associated with bacterial infections. *Salmonella sp, Escherichia coli, streptococcus fecalis, Staphylococcus aureus, Clostridia sp. (C. pefringens), Pseudomonas and Proteus spp.* have been isolated from cases of omphalitis. Chilling, overheating or stress during transport may predispose for the condition.

Inflammation of yolk sac, characterized by infected unhealed navels in young birds.

Clinical Signs

1. The affected newly hatched young are depressed, show drooping of the head and huddling near the heat source.
2. In many navel is seen inflamed and fails to close.
3. Edema and green, yellow discolouration of sternal subcutis may be seen.
4. Mortality often begins at hatching and continues up to 2 weeks age.
5. Omphalitis produce stunted birds.

Lesions

- The yolk sac is not absorbed and is congested (Figure 24).
- The yolk sac contents become watery and greenish yellow, occasionally, yolk contents become cheesy in appearance and consistency.
- Peritonitis may be present.

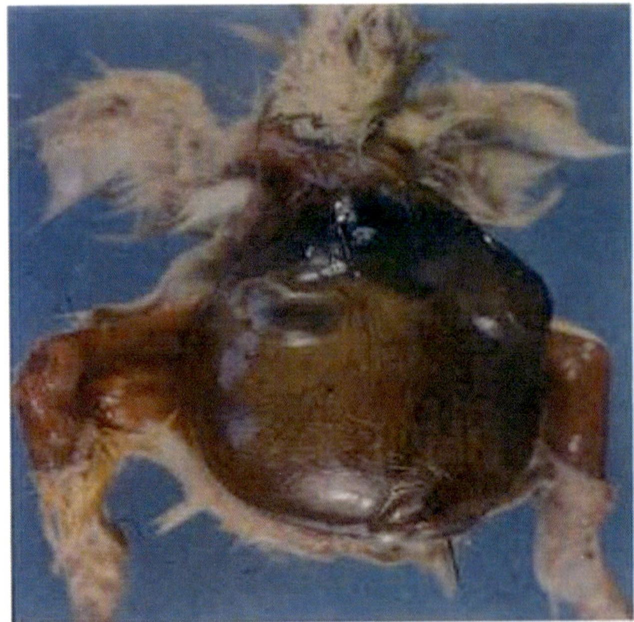

Fig. 24: Omphalitis (abdomen is greatly distended as a result of yolk sac infection)

Treatment

No specific treatment. Antibiotics may be useful. Identify the cause and remove it

Control

Sanitation in the incubator and maintenance of proper humidity and temperature in the brooding houses is helpful.

23

Staphylococcosis

The diseases caused by Staphylococci are found in all avian species and reported through out the world.

Etiology

There are more than 45 species and 25 subspecies in the genus Staphylococcus. *S. aureus* is the most common species of birds causing disease. Staphylococci are Gram - positive, coccoid and when grown on solid medium, bacteria form grape like clusters.

Transmission

Bacteria enter the body through skin wound or mucous membrane. It is more common in immunocompromised hosts., especially seen associated with Infectious bursal disease, Mareks' disease and Chicken infectious anaemia.

Clinical Signs

1) Affected birds initially show ruffled feathers, drooping of wings, lameness in one or both legs and fever.
2) These clinical signs are later seen progressing to severe depression swollen joints, reluctance to move and sitting on their hocks.
3) Morality and morbidity are low.

Lesions

1) Lesions of osteomyelitis mostly in the proximal end of tibiotarsus and femur are observed. Lesions of osteomyelitis may extend to distal part of tibiotarsus, femur, humerus, ribs and vertebrae.
2) Affected joints are swollen with inflammatory exudate.
3) Lesions of septicemia may develop which are seen as necrosis and congestion in visceral organs.
4) *S. aureus* is the main isolate from lesions of bumble foot (plantar abscess).

Diagnosis

Clinical signs are indicative of presumptive diagnosis. Isolation and identification of Staphylococci are recommended for the final diagnosis. Serology is not usually used in the diagnosis of this bacteria. PCR based molecular techniques are useful in the diagnosis.

Differential Diagnosis

Joint lesions caused by Staphylococcus aureus need be differentiated from *Salmonella pullorum/gallinarum, E. coli, Mycoplasma synovia, Pasteurella multocida and Reovirus* Which also produce similar lesions.

Treatment

S. aureus infection can be treated successfully with antimicrobial drugs.

Prevention and Control

In general, bacterins have been ineffective in poultry. In turkey, a live avirulent vaccine has been developed. The vaccine is given aerosol between 1-10 days, repeated at 4-6 weeks of age. Vaccine improved overall health and reduced the mortality. Similar results have been reported in chickens as well.

24

Streptococcus

Streptococcosis has been reported from avian species worldwide. Bacteria produce acute septicemic and chronic infection. Streptococcosis has wide range of host ranging from many avian species including wild birds.

Etiology

Streptococci are Gram-positive, non-spore forming, non-motile facultative anaerobes. They occur singly, in pairs or short chains. *S. zoozooepidemicus* is species associated with disease in avian species. Other species of streptococcus (*S. bovis, S. dysgalactiae, S. pleomorphus*) have occasionally been isolated from birds.

Transmission

Transmission occurs via oral and aerosol route.

Clinical Signs

1) The septicemic infection causes blood attained tissue and feathers around the head, yellow droppings, emaciation and anaemic comb and wattles.
2) There is egg drop in layers.
3) Mortality ranges from low to high (50%).

Lesions

1) In acute infection, hepatomegaly and splenomegaly with congestion and peritonitis of tissue are observed.
2) Blood stained tissue around the mouth and head.
3) Chronic infection is marked by fibrinous arthritis, tendosynovitis, osteomyelitis, perihepatitis, necrotic myocarditis and valvular endocarditis. Lesions of valvular endocarditis involve mostly mitral valves.

Diagnosis

Observation of Streptococci in blood smears, impression smears of lesions, especially from heart valve are diagnostic. Isolation and identification of Streptococci from lesions will confirm the diagnosis.

Latex agglutination test for the identification of Streptococci has been demonstrated.

Treatment

Antibiotics are useful in acute infection. In chronic form, efficacy of antibiotics decreases.

Prevention and Control

Proper cleaning and disinfection of premises help in prevention of the disease. Control of conditions causing immunosuppression helps in control.

25

Enterococcosis

Enterococcus sp. belongs to Lancefield antigenic serogroup *D. Enterococcus* is considered normal flora of the chicken intestine.

Etiology

Enterococci bacteria are Gram positive, spherical seen in singles, pairs or chain. *Enterococuus* sp. Causing disease in birds include *E. faecalis, E. faecium, E. durans, E. avium, E. hirae* and *E. cecorum. E. faecalis* is most common isolate from birds.

Transmission

Transmission occurs mainly through oral and aerosol route. Occasionally it infects birds through injured skin.

Clinical Signs

1) Disease caused by *E. faecalis* is in all age group. It is serious disease in embryos and young chicks which are infected through fecally contaminated eggs.
2) The disease is seen in 2 distinct forms: Acute and subacute/chronic form. In the acute form, clinical signs of septicemia are most prominent. They include depression, ruffled feathers, anaemia, diarrhoea and head tremors.
3) In layers, during acute disease, there is reduction in egg production.
4) In subacute and chronic form depression, lameness and head tremors are prominent clinical signs.

Lesions

1) Enlarged liver, kidney, spleen with congestion of subcutaneous tissue are observed in acute disease.
2) In subacute and chronic phase fibrinous arthritis, tendosynovitis, pericarditis and valvular endocarditis are main lesions.

Diagnosis

Demonstration of typical Enterococci in blood smears and impression smears from lesions may give tentative diagnosis. Speciation of Enterococci can be done through fermentation study of various sugar. Endocarditis caused by *Enterococcus fecalis* is also caused by many bacteria (*S. aureus, Strep. zooipedemicus, Past. multocida* and other species of Enterococci) hence isolation and identification of bacteria may assist in final diagnosis.

Treatment

Antibiotics are use full in treating the disease caused by Enterococci.

SECTION-3
Viral Diseases

26

Newcastle Disease (ND; Avian Pneumoencephalitis)

ND is a viral disease of poultry, wild and cage birds characterized by marked variation in morbidity, mortality, signs and lesions. Reported in 235 species of birds.

A disease of primary importance and concern worldwide which causes continuous massive economic loss. It is a reportable disease in many countries of the world.

Occurrence

Species: All birds susceptible. Temporary conjunctivitis may develop in people who come in close contact with NDV for the first time.

Etiology

Family Paramyxoviridae includes pathogenic viruses for animals, birds and man. It is divided into 2 subfamilies: Paramyxovirinae and Pneumovirinae. There are 11 serotypes of avian paramyxoviruses (APMV). APMV-1 serotype is Newcastle disease virus/Paramyxovirus Type 1 (NDV/PMV-1).

Epizootiology

1. Virus-containing excretions from infected birds including aerosols can contaminate feed, water, footwear, clothing, tools, equipment and the environment. Exposure of susceptible birds to any of these sources of the virus can result in transmission. Also, infected poultry may spread the virus if their tissues are used without proper processing in rendered products.
2. Eggs laid by infected hens may contain a virus; this could be a source of virus dissemination in a hatchery or layer unit.
3. Live virus vaccines may constitute a reservoir of NDV and chickens often shed the vaccine virus.

4. NDV can be introduced into a country by importing or smuggling of cage birds thereby transmitting the virus to poultry.
5. NDV has been isolated from sparrows, pigeons, doves, crows, owls and waterfowl. These birds may play a role in the spread of ND.

Pathogenesis

1. The disease produced following infection with NDV may vary considerably with the infecting virus.
2. The pathogenesis of NDV depends on some factors of which the most important are the virulence and tropism of the virus.
3. Other factors which may influence the morbidity, mortality and clinical signs are the host species, age, immune status, co-infection with other organisms, environmental stress, social stress, route of exposure, and the virus dose.
4. The virus varies widely on the type and severity of the disease that it produces. NDV strains can be divided into five pathotypes (Table 1) depending on the disease produced in chickens.

Clinical Signs

1. These are very variable depending on the strain of virus and the immune status of the flock. Acute and sub-acute strains cause respiratory signs, drops in egg production, soft shelled eggs, greenish loose faeces, and some torticollis or other nervous signs in individuals. Per-acute strains cause sudden death.
2. ND caused by lentogenic strains of the virus may produce few or no signs and little or no mortality.
3. ND caused by mesogenic strains of the virus is characterized by respiratory symptoms, concurrent or closely following CNS involvement and high mortality in younger birds; in layers, by a marked sudden drop in egg production, few or no signs and little or no mortality.
4. The velogenic form of ND is usually characterized by a short course, marked respiratory signs, diarrhoea and paralysis followed by the death of most affected birds.
5. In wild and cage birds, signs of ND include sudden deaths, gasping respiration, diarrhoea and later, the sign of CNS involvement.

Table 1: Newcastle disease virus (Avian paramyxovirus type 1 serotype) Pathotypes and the spectrum of disease

Pathotype	Clinical aspects	Lesions
Viscerotropic velogenic	Per acute systemic disease with > 90% mortality	Characteristic hemorrhagic lesion in the intestinal tract
Neurotropic velogenic	50-90% mortality following respiratory and nervous signs	Encephalitis dominant
Mesogenic	Respiratory disease followed by nervous signs with mortality up to 50%.	CNS involvement more in young chickens
Lentogenic	Mild or in apparent respiratory infection	Mild tracheitis to pneumonia
Asymptomatic	In apparent enteric infection	Negligible

Gross Lesions

1) Gastrointestinal tract (GIT)

- Hemorrhagic lesions of the intestinal tract, particularly the proventriculus (Figure 25), ceca, and small intestine (Figure 26).

2) Central nervous system (CNS)

- Gross lesions are not observed in the CNS of birds infected with NDV, regardless of the pathotype.

1. Respiratory tract

a. inflammation of the trachea, often with haemorrhages present

b. the air sacs may also be inflamed and appear cloudy and congested

2. Reproductive System

a. degeneration of follicles and atresia

b. resorption of yolk, congestion, haemorrhage and dark brown discolouration

c. oviducts shrunken and edematous

6. Skin and Eye

a. swelling of facial tissues and eyelids (oedema)

b. haemorrhage in conjunctivae

c. bleeding ulcers in the skin

Diagnosis

1) Epidemiological features.
2) Virus isolation and identification.
3) Serology
    a. Hemagglutination (HA) and Hemagglutination inhibition (HI) tests with the virus. Rising titers to HI test or ELISA.
    b. Virus neutralization test using known NDV antiserum
    c. Plaque neutralization test in a tissue culture system
4) Inoculation of the virus into known-immune and known-susceptible chickens

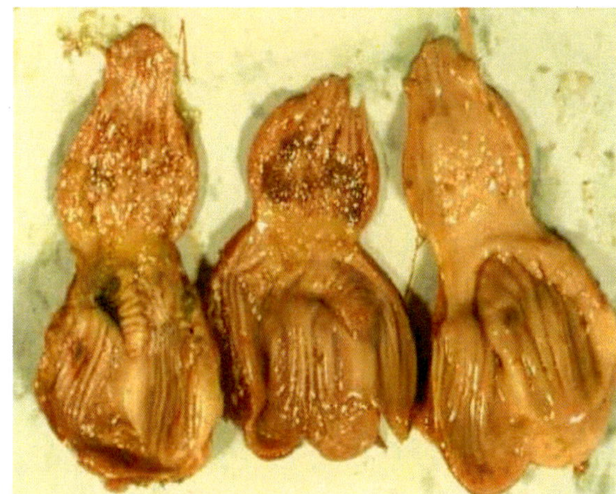

Fig. 25: Newcastle disease; Hemorrhages in the proventriculus,

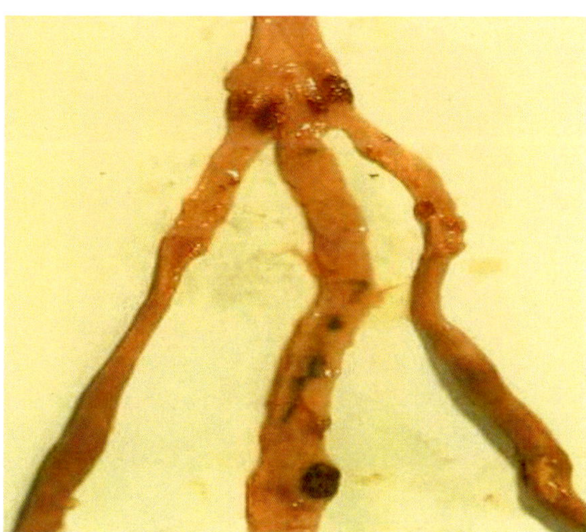

Fig. 26: Newcastle disease; Hemorrhages in the cecal tonsils and intestinal mucosa.

5) Fluorescent antibody technique using a conjugated NDV antiserum
6) Immunohistochemistry for detection of viral antigens in tissues
7) PCR based molecular techniques

Differential Diagnosis

Avian influenza, Avian encephalomyelitis, Infectious bronchitis, Infectious laryngotracheitis, Marek's disease, encephalomalacia

Prevention and Control

• Immediate Action

1) Quarantine up to a radius of 5 Km from the focus of outbreak.
2) Vaccination of susceptible birds within the quarantine area. The live vaccine can be used in the face of an outbreak, in nearby unvaccinated stocks as well.
3) Destruction of affected birds with immediate disinfection and quarantine measures.

• Long Term Action

1) Follow proper vaccination schedules. Raise vaccinated birds. Effective vaccines are available.
2) Control imports of poultry, poultry products and cage birds.

Treatment

Treatment of ND is of no value.

27

Pneumovirus Infections (Turkey Rhinotracheitis, TRT and Swollen Head Syndrome, SHS)

Etiology

The subfamily Pneumovirinae includes two genera: Pneumoviruses and metapneumovirus. The later consists of both human and avian metapneumovirus (aMPV). aMPV produces turkey rhinotracheitis (TRT) in turkey and Swollen head syndrome (SHS) in chickens. aMPV has been detected in other species of birds, but the disease in those birds are not well defined.

Occurrence Species

A new disease of turkeys (in the UK since 1985) which is suspected to cause some lesser problems in chickens.

Age Rang

a) **TRT:** Any age may be affected.

b) **SHS:** Affects mainly 4-6 week old broilers, but also occasionally observed in broiler breeder.

Transmission and Epizootiology

1) Contact transmission from affected to susceptible turkey poults and chicks by inoculation with filtered or unfiltered mucus, nasal washings, or other materials from the respiratory tract of affected birds.

2) Contaminated water, movement of affected or recovered turkey and chicken, movement of personnel and equipment, feed, trucks, etc. have been implicated in some outbreaks.

3) Airborne or vertical transmission is also possible. The air borne spread is rapid.

4) Contaminated water, movement of affected or recovered poults, movement of personnel and equipment, feed, trucks, etc. have been implicated in some outbreaks.

Clinical Signs

a) TRT

1) Turkeys develop a sudden respiratory disease with ocular and nasal discharges and distension of the infraorbital sinus.
2) Signs in young poults include snicking, rales, sneezing, frothy nasal discharge, foamy conjunctivitis, swelling of the infraorbital sinuses, and submandibular oedema.
3) A temporary drop in egg production in laying turkeys.
4) The virus is immunosuppressive and secondary bacterial/fungal infections of the lungs occur if ventilation/husbandry is defective.

b) SHS

1) In chickens, temporary depression, reduced egg production and lung/air sac lesions reported from the field (swollen head in broilers may be associated with this infection).
2) Signs in broiler breeders include swelling of the periorbital and infraorbital sinuses, swelling of lacrimal glands, sneezing, torticollis, cerebral disorientation, depression and variable mortality.
3) Egg production losses are also associated with SHS.
4) In chickens, E coli in association with aMPV may cause SHS.

Lesions

• Gross

1) No specific lesions - various respiratory lesions.
2) Petechiation to severe congestion of the turbinate mucosa and lacrimal glands
3) Purulent and edematous subcutaneous cellulitis in SHS

Diagnosis / Sampling

1) Clinical signs and epidemiology of outbreak.
2) Virus isolation in tissue culture.

3) Serological tests are being developed (ELISA and VN tests).
4) Immunofluorescence and immunodiffusion tests.
5) PCR based molecular techniques

Differential Diagnosis

Because of similar signs and lesions produced by other bacteria (Bordetella species which causes turkey coryza, and mycoplasma gallisepticum;) and many viruses (Newcastle disease virus, Infectious bronchitis virus and influenza viruses) differentiation of these conditions need to be made for a conclusive diagnosis.

Specimens Required

1) Affected live birds
2) Nasal secretions or tissue scraped from the sinuses of affected birds.
3) Serum from the flock

Prevention and Control

• Immediate Action

Clinical judgment will determine if anti-bacterial medication required in mild cases, it is of doubtful value.

Long Term Vaccination

Live attenuated, and inactivated aMPV vaccines are commercially being used with limited success. Occasionally reversion of vaccine to the virulent strain of aMPV has been reported.

Treatment

Antibiotic therapy has met with varied success.

28

Infectious Laryngotracheitis (Laryngotracheitis, ILT; LT)

ILT is an acute viral disease of chickens, pheasants and peafowl characterized by marked dyspnea, coughing, gasping and expectoration of bloody exudate. The disease is worldwide.

Hosts

Chickens particularly susceptible; reported to occur in pheasants and peafowl.

Age Range

All ages susceptible but is most often found in adult (mature or nearly mature) commercial chicken layers.

Etiology

Gallid herpes virus Type 1 of the herpesviridae family.

Epizootiology

1) Some recovered chickens and vaccinated chickens become carriers and shed virus for long periods of time, thus exposing other susceptible birds.
2) Mechanical transmission of the virus via fomites is also possible.
3) The disease spreads laterally after it has been introduced, although the spread is less rapid than with other viral respiratory diseases of chickens.

Clinical Signs

1) Enzootic mild forms (Strains of low pathogenicity)

Conjunctivitis, lacrimation, nasal discharge, swollen infraorbital sinuses, and lowered egg production with very few deaths (0.2%) from upper tracheal obstruction.

2) Acute disease (High pathogenic strains)

a. Marked dyspnea with gasping and coughing; in severity, chickens raise and extend their head and neck during inspiration (Figure 27) making loud wheezing sounds.

b. Expectoration of bloody mucus consequent to coughing and head shaking; beaks, faces or feathers of some birds may be bloody.

c. High morbidity and considerable mortality (10-40%).

Lesions

1) Tracheal epithelium inflamed and may be desquamated resulting in plugs which occlude the larynx and cause asphyxiation.

2) Haemorrhage in the trachea in severe cases (Figure 28).

3) Infected birds often have a bloody beak or blood on the face, head or feathers.

Diagnosis

1) History and typical clinical signs;

2) Histopathology (I/N inclusions in the epithelial cells of trachea (Figure 29) and conjunctiva during early stages of the disease)

3) Virus isolation and tissue culture

4) FAT

5) Exposure of known-immune and known susceptible chickens to the virus.

6) Serology (ELISA, VN)

7) Electron microscopy

8) PCR based molecular techniques

Differential Diagnosis

Avian influenza, Infectious bronchitis, Mycoplasmosis.

Prevention and Control

1) Eradication from the site: contaminated premises should be depopulated, cleaned, disinfected and left vacant for 4-6 weeks before being used again.

2) Routine vaccination of young stock [4-12 weeks] with live vaccines (eye drop and other routes [drinking water, aerosol spray]) is required.

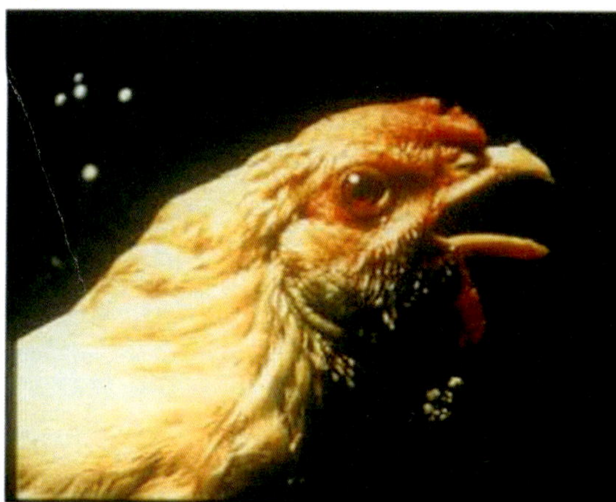

Fig. 27: ILT; Chicken showing difficult breathing.

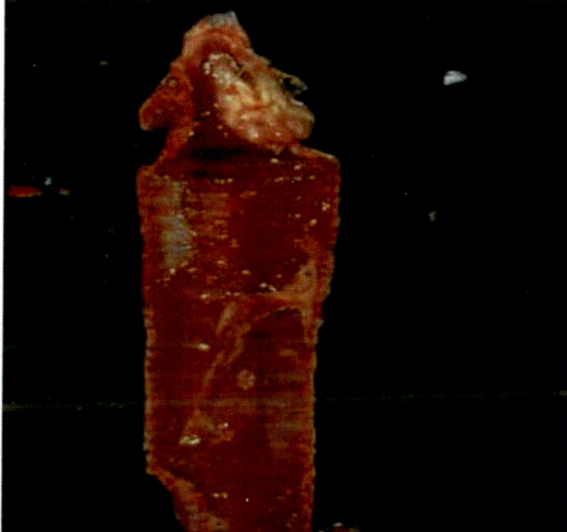

Fig. 28: ILT; Acute form, hemorrhagic trachea.

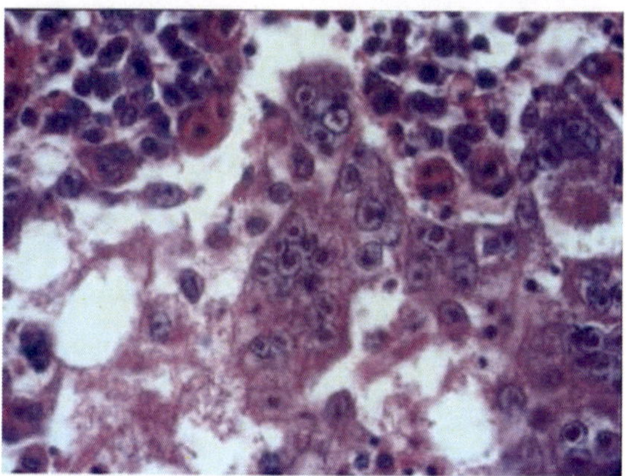

Fig. 29: ILT; Intra-nuclear inclusions seen in the sloughed epithelial cells of the trachea

3) Avoid adding vaccinated, recovered or exposed birds to a susceptible flock and maintain strict quarantine measures.

Treatment

Treatment is of little or no value.

29

Infectious Bronchitis (IB)

IB is an acute, highly contagious, viral disease of chickens characterized by respiratory signs (gasping, sneezing, coughing, and nasal discharge), the severe renal disease associated with neurotropic strains, and a marked decrease in egg production. It is a serious cause of sub-optimal egg production and poor egg quality. This disease is worldwide in ditribution.

Hosts

Chickens only. Recently IBV has been detected in species other than chickens. The disease may be produced only in chickens, IBV may multiply in other species of birds and be a source of infection.

Etiology

IB is caused by the avian coronavirus; numerous strains of infectious bronchitis virus (IBV) exist because of high genetic diversity and cross protection between strains is not reliable.

Epizootiology

1) Transmission of IB is by inhalation or ingestion of virus-containing droplets expelled by infected, coughing chickens.
2) Transmission may also occur by virus infected fomites, tools, clothing etc. contaminated with the virus.
3) Aerosol transmission occurs over considerable distance and morbidity is very high.

Clinical Signs

The incubation period is short (18 to 36 hours). All birds in the flock become infected, but mortality is observed only in young chicks, which may be as high as 25% and is negligible in chickens over six weeks of age. Mortality depends on the virulence of the virus strain and age of the chickens. The Australian T strain causes greater mortality in chicks.

A. In young chicks

1) Mainly respiratory signs: gasping, coughing, tracheal rales and nasal discharge.

2) The eyes are wet, and a few chicks may have swollen sinuses. (Figure 30).

B. In growing chicks over 5-6 weeks of age

1) The clinical signs include tracheal rales, gasping and coughing.

2) However, the respiratory symptoms are not severe and may not be noticed unless carefully observed.

C. In adult laying flocks

1) **Respiratory signs:** Gasping, coughing and tracheal rales seen for a short period.

2) There is a drop in egg production, which varies with the time of lay. Flocks infected in the early part of laying suffer only a slight drop returning to normal level in a few weeks. Flocks infected in the latter half of their laying period usually have a severe drop in egg production. Such flocks take a long time to recover to normal production.

3) Accompanying a drop in egg production, there may be soft-shelled, misshapen and rough-shelled eggs. Shell irregularities usually remain for a longer period.

4) Internal quality of eggs is also affected. The albumen is thin, watery and lack demarcation between thick and thin albumen (Figure 31).

Gross Lesions

1) Where the clinical signs are mainly respiratory, lesions are mainly in the upper respiratory tract. These include serous or catarrhal exudate in the trachea, nasal passages and sinuses. In complicated cases, lesions of the airsac disease may develop.

2) Reproductive tract lesions include a reduction in length and weight of the oviduct. However, it returns to normal in 3-4 weeks of recovery.

3) Chicks infected in the early part of their life develop permanent damage to the oviduct. The magnum and isthmus become hypoplastic, followed by normal growth of the oviduct adjacent to the affected part; it causes cystic oviduct. Such birds become internal layers.

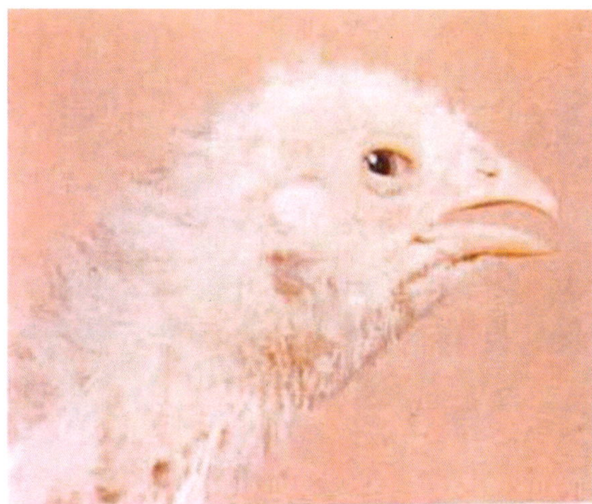

Fig. 30: IB; Chick breathing through mouth as a result of swollen sinuses,

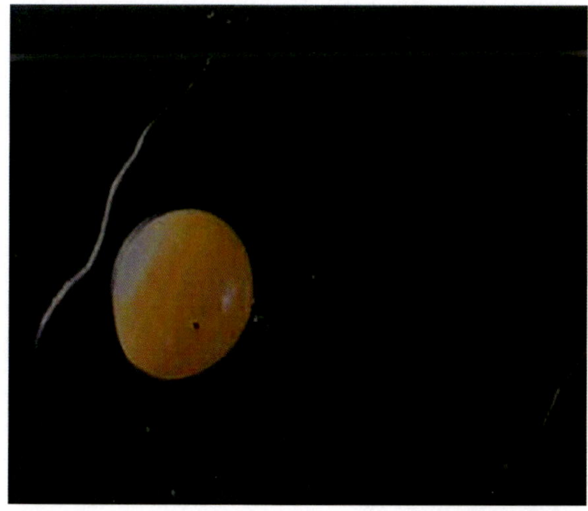

Fig. 31: IB; Changes in the internal quality of egg; albumen becomes watery.

4) Severe kidney lesions with certain IBV strains include swelling and pale discolouration of the kidneys and occlusion of the ureters with uric acid.

Diagnosis

1) Clinical and epidemiological signs.

2) Virus isolation in 9-12 day-old chicken embryos. Many passages are required before a conclusion is made. The constant lesions within seven days of inoculation of IBV are death, stunting of embryos and urate deposition in kidneys.

3) **Serology:** rising titer to SN, HI or ELISA tests.

4) Inoculation of IB immune and IB susceptible chicks with the isolated virus; in susceptible chicks, clinical signs of respiratory distress develop within 48 hours.

5) Detection of viral antigens in tissue (trachea, kidneys) by FAT and immunohistochemistry.

6) PCR based molecular techniques to classify the strains based on genotype.

Differential Diagnosis

IB may resemble those diseases where respiratory signs are observed. These are Newcastle disease, Infectious laryngotracheitis, Infectious coryza, Avian influenza, and Mycoplasmosis. Drop in egg production should be differentiated from Egg drop syndrome and mineral deficiency.

ND may be differentiated from IB by

1) The severity of disease; ND is more severe causing mortality in all age groups.

2) Presence of nervous signs in young chicks in ND.

3) Egg drop in layers is severe in ND.

ILT may be differentiated from IB by

1) Morbidity; ILT spreads slowly, and lesions are severe.

2) There is a hemorrhagic tracheitis in ILT.

3) ILT does not affect younger birds.

Infectious coryza can be differentiated from IB by the presence of facial swelling and bad odour in the flock.

Prevention and Control

Vaccination

1) Chicks that have recovered from the natural disease are resistant to homologous strains of the virus for at least a year.
2) Chicks hatched from recovered and immunized hens carry antibodies for up to 4 weeks; however, these antibodies do not prevent respiratory infection, although they may affect the severity of the disease.
3) Live and inactivated vaccines are available; mainly two serotypes (Massachusetts and Connecticut types) are used in a vaccine. Lack of cross protection between serotypes of vaccine and the field can be one of the explanations for "vaccine break" in IB.
4) Chicks in the high-risk area should be vaccinated at day-old or delayed for up to 7-21 days. Route of vaccination can be eye drop, nasal drop, coarse spray or drinking water.
5) Layers and breeder chickens should be revaccinated at 16-18 weeks of age with inactivated IB vaccine (oil emulsion) by injection for longer protection.

Treatment

No effective treatment of IB is known although antibiotics may control the complications.

30

Infectious Anemia (Chicken Anemia Agent [CAA] infection)

This 'virus' is widespread in commercial flocks worldwide, but its taxonomic position is not determined. The disease is characterized by aplastic anaemia and generalized lymphoid atrophy with a concomitant immunosuppression. Consequently, infectious anaemia is frequently complicated by viral, bacterial, or fungal infections.

Occurrence

Chickens up to 3 weeks of age are most susceptible.

Etiology

A small DNA virus called Chicken Infectious Anemia Virus (CIAV). Representative isolate is called "Del-Ros strain". Similar pathogenic but antigenically distinct strains from CIAV are being isolated. The virus has not yet been classified; it shares characteristics of porcine circovirus and psittacine beak and feather virus (a circovirus). It is being proposed to put all three together.

Transmission

1) Primary transmission is vertical. It occurs when negative antibody hens become infected.
2) Horizontal:When a high concentration of virus is present in faeces for 5-7 weeks after infection. Horizontal transmission occurs by direct and indirect contact- oral-faecal route.

Clinical Signs

1) The specific sign is hemorrhagic aplastic anaemia syndrome - hematocrit values range from 6% to 27% (normal 35%) (Figure 32) seen mainly in 2-3 week old chicks. Low hematocrit values are due to pancytopenia, decreased number of RBC, WBC and thrombocytes. Decreased clotting and haemorrhages are the sequel of thrombocytopenia.

2) Non -specific signs- Depression, decreased weight gain and pale tissues.
3) Mortality is between 5 and 10%, rising to 60% in complicated cases.
4) The virus causes concomitant immunosuppression, hence frequently complicated with bacterial, viral and mycotic infections.

Gross Lesions

1) Thymic atrophy (Figure 33) and bone marrow hypoplasia (Figure 34, 35).
2) Subcutaneous, muscular, mucosal or sub serosal haemorrhages.

   Hemorrhages in proventriculus are significant for the differential with NCD.
3) Atrophy of the bursa of Fabricius.
4) Swelling and mottled appearance of the liver.
5) Lesions of secondary bacterial infections like dermatitis.

Diagnosis

1) Virus isolation and identification.
2) Serology is useful in flock survey

Differential Diagnosis

1) The diseases causing atrophy of lymphoid tissues (Marek's disease, Gumboro disease)
2) The diseases causing aplastic anaemia and hemorrhagic syndrome (intoxications, sulfonamides, mycotoxins).

Prevention and Control

Vaccination of breeder pullets at about 16-18 weeks of age, by injection or drinking water. Results of vaccinations are variable.

Treatment

There is no effective treatment for this condition.

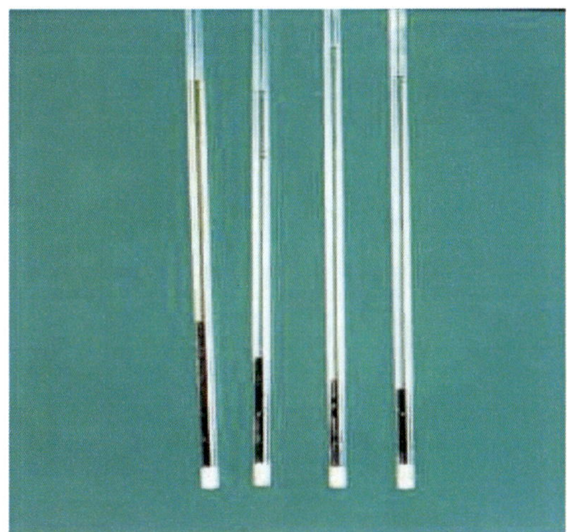

Fig. 32: Chicken infectious anemia virus infection; low hematocrit value in infected chicken

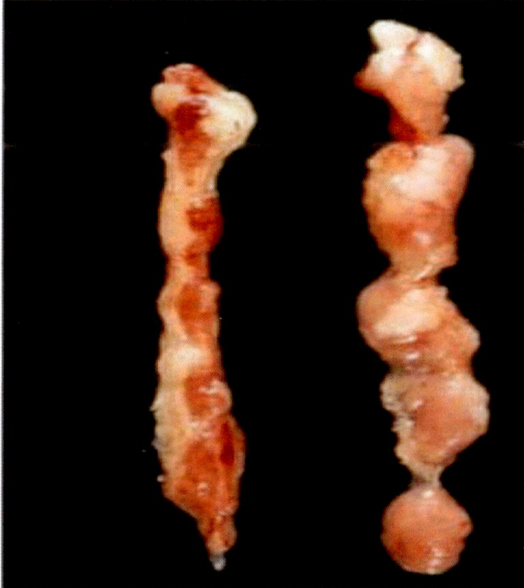

Fig. 33: CIAV infection; severe atrophy of thymus compared to normal thymus at the right,

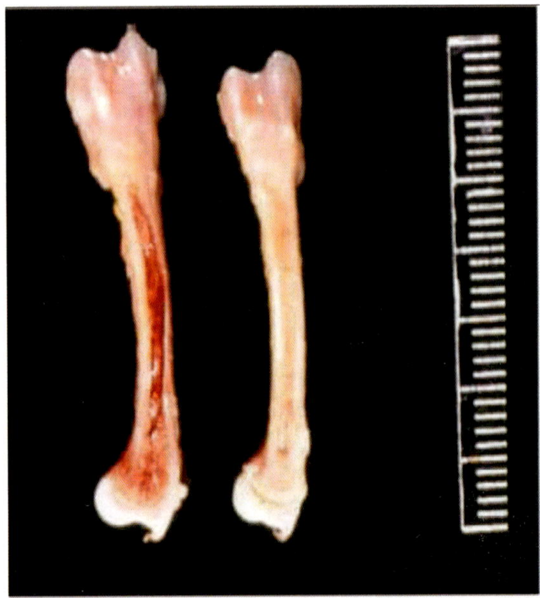

Fig. 34: CIAV infection; pale yellow fatty marrow (right) compared to normal marrow

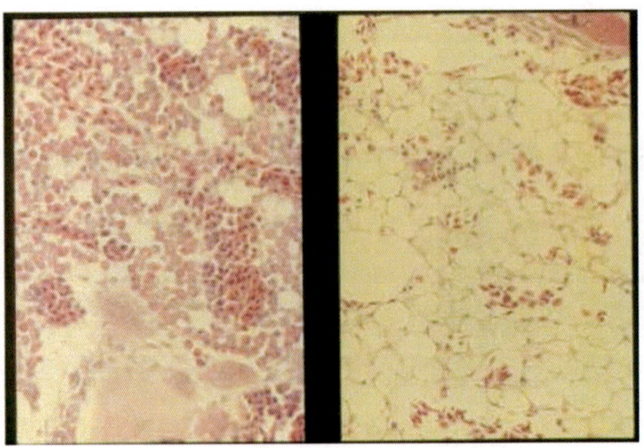

Fig. 35: CIAV infection; severe hypoplasia of erythroid and myeloid cells and replacement by adipose tissue, compared to normal on the left.

31

Adenovirus Infections of Chickens

Adenoviruses have been found in several species of birds and animals. There are at least 12 serotypes of chicken adenoviruses. The chicken adenoviruses are host specific, meaning they will not infect other animal species. Avian adenoviruses are divided into three major groups. Members of each type may share group antigens, but there is no common antigen shared between types.

Classification

- **Group 1 (aviadenovirus)** includes Quail Bronchitis, hydropericardium, Gizzard erosions and Inclusion body hepatitis agent;
- **Group II (Siaadenovirus)** causes marble spleen disease in pheasants and Hemorrhagic enteritis in turkeys and splenomegaly in chickens.
- **Group III (adenovirus)** causes Egg drop syndrome.

Transmission

1) through embryos – vertical
2) through faeces – horizontal through contamination of feed, water and fomites (2-3 week after infection). Shedding of virus in faeces and through embryos stops with the development of antibody.

32

Quail Bronchitis (QB)

Quail bronchitis (QB) is caused by group I (aviadenovirus). QB is an acute respiratory disease of bobwhite quail, occasionally with high mortality. Disease has sporadic occurrence many parts of the world. QB virus is closely related to the prototype CELO (chick embryo lethal orphan) virus, which is cause of high mortality in chicks.

Transmission

Although not well understood, transmission is suspected through aerosol.

Clinical Signs

The disease is severe in quails up to 6 weeks age and sub clinical in older quails. Quails show tracheal rales, coughing, sneezing and conjunctivitis. A few may have nervous signs.

Mortality varies between 10 and 100%.

Lesions

Tracheal and bronchial mucosa is inflamed with mucus inflammation. Air sacs may be cloudy.

Diagnosis

1) Acute onset with high mortality in young quails.
2) Presence of intranuclear inclusions in respiratory epithelium.
3) Isolation and identification of virus in cell cultures and chicken embryos.
4) Agar gel precipitation test for type -I adenovirus.

Prevention and Control

The breeding flocks should be kept free of infection. The quail flocks kept away from chicken flocks.

No vaccine is available.

There is no effective treatment.

33

Inclusion Body Hepatitis (IBH; Adenoviral Infection)

IBH is an adenovirus infection of young chickens characterized by sudden onset and sharply increased mortality, short course, anaemia, and hepatitis often accompanied by intranuclear inclusion bodies. It is described in Canada, USA and many other countries.

Occurrence

- Species: **Chickens only (broilers and pullets).**
- Age Range: **3-15 week old chickens but more frequently in 4-8 week old chickens.**

Etiology

1) Avian adenovirus group I.
2) Predisposing factors
3) Immunosuppressive effects of early IBD

Epizootiology

1) Infected chickens eliminate adenovirus in their faeces for a few weeks, and thus infection can spread slowly through a flock.
2) The virus is resistant to many environmental influences and can spread readily on fomites or mechanically.
3) The virus can be transmitted through the egg.
4) Lateral spread of virus occurs through contaminated feed, water and environment.

Clinical Signs

1) Sudden marked increase in mortality for 3-5 days, levelling off for 3-5 days and then decreasing to normal levels over 3-5 days. Total mortality may approach 10%.
2) Morbidity is low and affected chicks show signs for only a few hours and then die.
3) Depression, listlessness, pallor of comb, wattles and facial skin are the main clinical signs.

Lesions Gross

1) Pallor and icterus of skin with haemorrhages particularly over the legs and breast.
2) Haemorrhages in skeletal muscles and under serous membranes.
3) Swelling of the liver which may be yellow to tan in colour with parenchymal and capsular petechiae and ecchymoses.
4) Pale swollen kidneys with cortical haemorrhages.
5) Bone marrow is pale yellow, and blood is thin and watery.
6) Atrophy of the bursa of Fabricius and spleen.

Histopathology

1) Extensive degeneration and necrosis of the liver with intranuclear inclusions in hepatocytes during the early stages of the disease.
2) Hypoplasia of the bone marrow.

Diagnosis

1) Sudden increase in mortality with low morbidity in young growing flocks.
2) Histopathological demonstration of lesions in liver with presence of intranuclear inclusions in hepatocytes.
3) Virus isolation
4) Agar gel precipitation test

Prevention and Control

No vaccine is available

Treatment

1) There is no effective treatment for chickens with IBH.
2) Good husbandry and care usually suppress mortality.

34

Hydropericardium Syndrome (HS)

Etiology

Group 1 adenovirus. First reported in Pakistan in 1987, where it caused a devastating effect on broiler industry. It has spread to all continents.

Transmission

Spread vertically and horizontally.

Clinical Signs and Lesions

1) Mortality starts at three weeks, peaks for 4-8 days and then decline. Mortality ranges between 20% and 80%. Adult birds also show the disease but with low mortality.
2) Clear straw coloured flued accumulates in the pericardial sac, and in lungs.
3) Liver and kidneys are enlarged.

Diagnosis

Isolation and identification of aviadenovirus from faeces and affected tissues/ organs. Confirmation of isolates can be made through electron microscopy and PCR. Serology is also helpful.

NECROTIZING PANCREATITIS AND GIZZARD EROSION

The condition is described in broiler chickens. The slight losses in weight and low mortality have been found in many flocks. However, in the absence of specific clinical signs and lesions, the condition is mostly observed at the slaughter house / necropsy table. The gizzard is distended with hemorrhagic fluid. Black patchy erosions are noted in the gizzard kaolin layer. Experimental inoculation of virus in young broilers produced lesions 3 - 18 days PI. Diagnosis is confirmed on specific lesions in gizzard and pancreas and isolation/identification of the virus.

35

EGG Drop Syndrome 1976 (EDS 76)

EDS 76 is an infectious disease of laying hens caused by hemagglutinating adenovirus and characterized by failure to achieve production targets or by the production of thin-shelled or shell-less eggs in otherwise healthy birds.

This important disease caused loss of egg production for several years - vaccination introduced the disease and a new vaccine virtually eradicated it.

Occurrence

Chickens (laying hens) although the causative virus has been recovered from ducks, geese and other waterfowls

Etiology

Group III adenovirus. It is also called EDS 76 virus since it was diagnosed in 1976 causing the drop in egg production - this adenovirus of duck origin was introduced into poultry flocks via a contaminated live vaccine in 1976.

Epizootiology

1) Initially, there is a vertical transmission from breeders to progeny; virus remains latent until birds approached peak production when the virus is excreted, and spread of virus occurs.
2) Lateral spread occurs through contact with infected faeces. During viremic stage, virus is shed in faeces and from the pharynx. Eggs laid during the period of "egg drop" contain virus on its interior and exterior. This leads to contamination of egg trays.
3) Infected chicken develops viremia, and mechanical transmission of the virus can occur through contaminated needles.
4) Natural transmission of the virus from ducks and other waterfowl to chickens through drinking water contaminated by droppings occurs occasionally.

Clinical Signs

1) Layers from 26-35 weeks of age are more affected.
2) The most important sign is a drop in laying. Eggs produced during the "laying drop" show poor egg- shell quality (production of thin-shelled or shell-less eggs) and colour (loss of colour in pigmented eggs); (Figure 36).
3) The disease spreads slowly in the flock. This character differentiates it from other diseases, which affect laying – such as IB, and ND. Laying drop is usually for 6-12 weeks, after which it comes to normal.

   This leads to a period of erratic egg production followed by recovery.
4) Drop in egg production of up to 40% have been described.

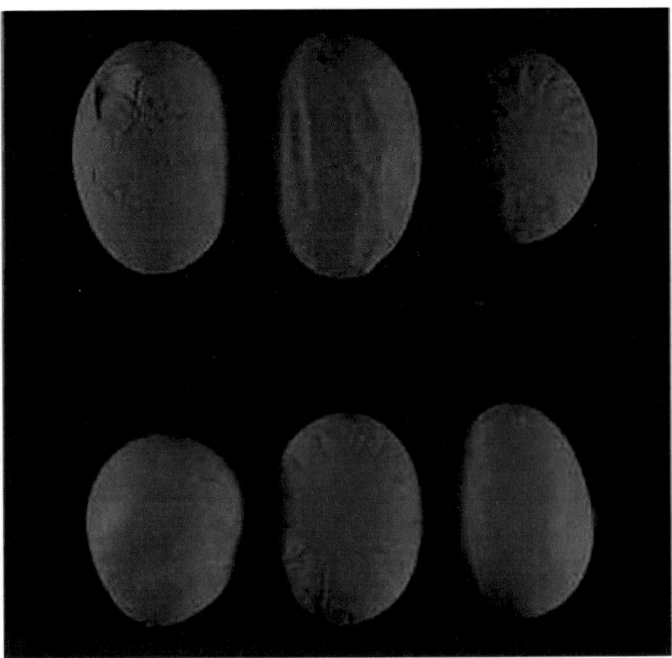

Fig. 36: Egg drop syndrome; Irregularly shaped, soft shelled or shell less eggs

Gross Lesions

There are no gross lesions although some times uterine oedema has been observed in experimental infections.

Diagnosis

1) Reduction in production with the occurrence of depigmented, soft-shelled eggs in the absence of other clinical signs should trigger consideration of EDS 76.
2) Serology: HI, ELISA, SN, FA and DID tests. HI, and SN tests are flock tests most helpful in sero- diagnosis.
3) Virus isolation: Best achieved in embryonated duck or goose eggs or cell culture of duck or goose origin. No growth has been detected in chicken eggs.
4) FAT with labelled EDS antiserum used in cell cultures.
5) PCR based molecular techniques

Prevention and Control

Vaccinate before start of egg production (at 14-16 weeks of age). An effective inactivated vaccine is available; 0.5 ml of the vaccine is injected subcutaneously or intramuscularly.

Treatment

There is no successful treatment.

36

Viral Arthritis

(Tenosynovitis; Ruptured gastrocnemius tendon; Reovirus infection)

Viral arthritis is a reovirus infection primarily of broilers characterized by arthritis and tenosynovitis (primarily of the tarsus and metatarsus, the digital flexor and tarsometatarsal extensor tendons) and, occasionally, by rupture of the gastrocnemius tendon(s) resulting in lameness and condemnations at slaughter. The disease is reported worldwide.

Occurrence

Chickens only (broilers) but the virus has been found in higher breeds of chicken and turkeys. 4-16 week old birds are more susceptible.

Etiology

A reovirus which is quite resistant to many environmental factors.

Epizootiology

Reovirus is discharged in faeces of infected chickens suggesting faecal contamination as the primary source of horizontal transmission.Virus in infected faeces may contaminate eggshells and transmitted vertically.

Clinical Signs

1) Lameness and swelling of the tendon sheaths of the shanks and the gastrocnemius tendon above the hock are early signs. Affected chickens prefer to sit and reluctant to move (Figure 37).
2) Shanks of affected chickens are enlarged.
3) Rupture of the gastrocnemius tendon results in immobilization, unthriftiness and stunting of affected birds.

Gross Lesions

1) Swelling and inflammation of the tendons and tendon sheaths above the hock (Figure 38) and rupture of gastrocnemius tendon (Figure 39). The affected joint contains an Excess of lemon yellow to brownish blood tinged or occasionally purulent exudate.

2) Hemorrhage in the tendons and erosions on the synovial membranes of the articular cartilages of the hock. In chronic cases, fibrosis and adhesions of affected tendons may occur.

Diagnosis

1) History and signs of bilateral enlargement of the tendon sheaths of the shanks.

2) Histopathological confirmation of tenosynovitis.

3) FAT

4) Agar gel precipitin test

5) Virus isolation

6) PCR base techniques for identification of the virus

Differential Diagnosis

Causes of lameness and lesions of arthritis must be differentiated from other conditions like mycoplasmosis, bacterial arthritis, salmonellosis, Marek's disease, pasteurellosis, deformities and nutritional diseases. Dual infections can exist.

Prevention and Control

Vaccination of breeder flocks for transfer of maternal antibodies to their progeny. Age associated resistance develops after two weeks. A viable attenuated strain of isolate has been used as a commercial vaccine for broiler breeders; the vaccine is given during 10-15 weeks of age in drinking water.

Vaccination of 1-day-old chicks, obtained from unvaccinated breeders can be by spray or subcutaneous injection. Vaccine interferes with Marek's disease vaccination given by injection.

Treatment

There is no satisfactory treatment.

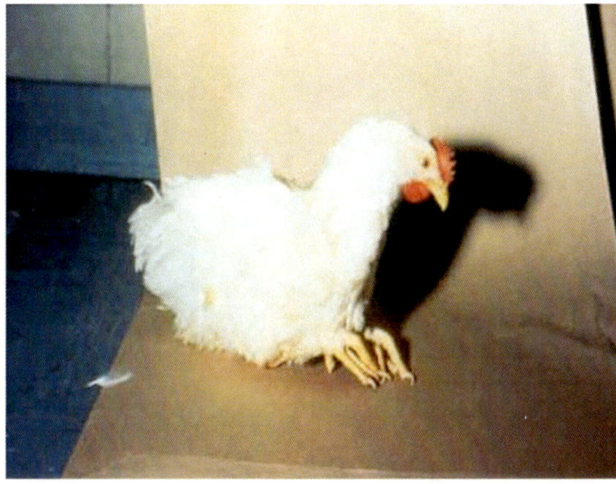

Fig. 37: Viral arthritis; Chicken with tendo-sinovitis, prefers to sit and reluctant to move

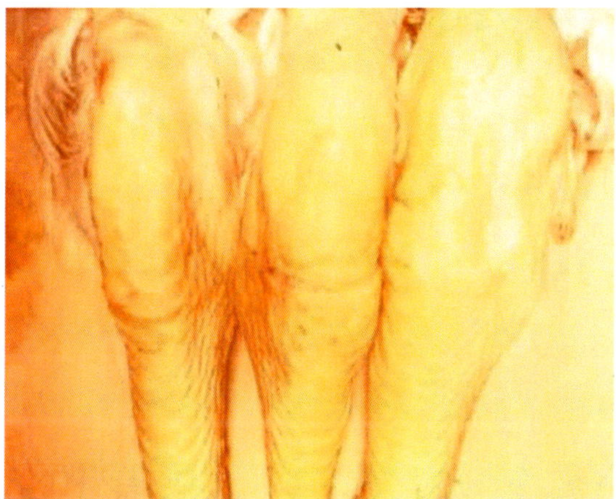

Fig. 38: Viral arthritis; Swelling of tendon sheath above the hock joint- a characteristic lesion;

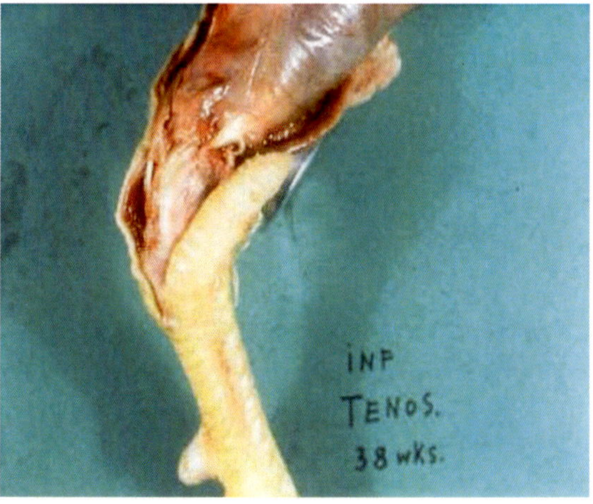

Fig. 39: Viral arthritis; Rupture of gastrocnemius tendon

37

Fowl Pox (Pox; Avian Pox)

Fowl pox is a slow spreading viral disease of chickens, turkeys and other birds characterized by cutaneous lesions on the un-feathered skin of the head, neck, legs and feet and/or by diphtheritic lesions in the upper digestive and respiratory tract. The disease is worldwide in distribution.

Occurrence

Among poultry chicken and turkey are more susceptible. Other birds include pigeons, canaries, psittacines and wild birds. Fowl pox has been reported from more than 200 species of birds. The incidence is severe in multiple age groups and intensive poultry farming areas.

Etiology

Pox virus (avian type) belongs to Avipox virus genus in poxviridae family. Strains of the virus exist: fowl pox, pigeon pox, canary pox, turkey pox and quail pox. Serologically strains cross react but antigenic and immunologic differences exist.

Epizootiology

Virus-containing crusts (scabs) formed on the skin are desquamated into the litter.

Virus persists in the environment and may later infect susceptible birds by entering the skin through minor abrasions and respiratory route.

Mosquitoes transmit the virus within the flock and from farm to farm.

Clinical Signs

a) Cutaneous Form

Predominates in most outbreaks and affects the featherless parts of the head, comb, wattles, corner of mouth, angle of beak and around eyelids (Figure 40) and foot.

b) Diphtheritic Form

1) Seen in mouth, nares, larynx, pharynx, oesophagus and trachea (Figure 41).
2) Diphtheritic lesions in the upper respiratory or digestive tract may result in dyspnea or inappetance respectively.
3) Lesions in the nasal cavity or conjunctiva lead to nasal or ocular discharge.
4) Extension of lesions to infraorbital sinuses produce coryza like lesions.
5) Mortality usually low depending on the virulence of the strain and intercurrent infection. In young chickens and turkeys, it ranges 10% to 20%.rising to 50% in severe cases.

c) Systemic Disease

Common in canaries and finches. Pox in canaries is usually fatal.

Gross Lesions

1) Cutaneous lesions usually occur on the unfeathered skin of the head and neck but may take place around the vent or on the feet or legs.
2) Hyperplasia of the epithelium leading to the formation of papules, vesicles, pustules or crusts (scabs) which may coalesce - lesions eventually heal.
3) Diphtheritic lesions are raised yellow plaques on mucous membranes predominating in the mouth but may be present in the sinuses, nasal cavity, conjunctiva, pharynx, larynx, trachea or oesophagus.
4) Systemic disease is common in Finches and canaries, marked by hepatomegaly and splenomegaly, with lesions in the oral cavity and respiratory tract. Liver and spleen are enlarged by infiltration of immature lymphoid cells.

Diagnosis

1) Clinical signs may be diagnostic.
2) Histopathologically, intracytoplasmic inclusions (Bollinger bodies) can be demonstrated in the infected epithelium.
3) Inoculation of suspected material into chicken embryos. Typical pocks develop on the chorio -allantoic membrane.
4) PCR based molecular technique

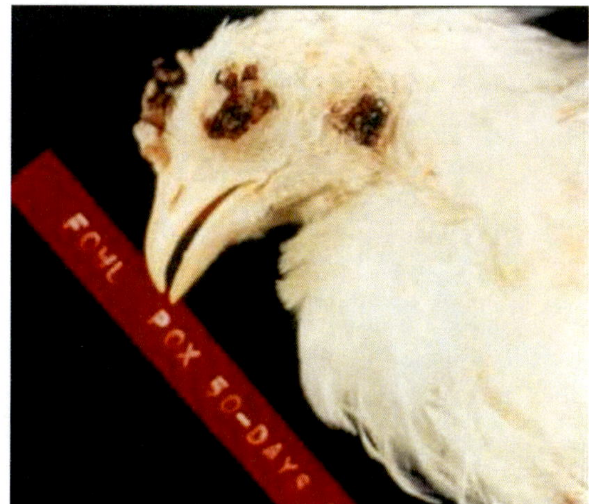

Fig.40: Fowl pox; Cutaneous lesions on comb and eye lids;

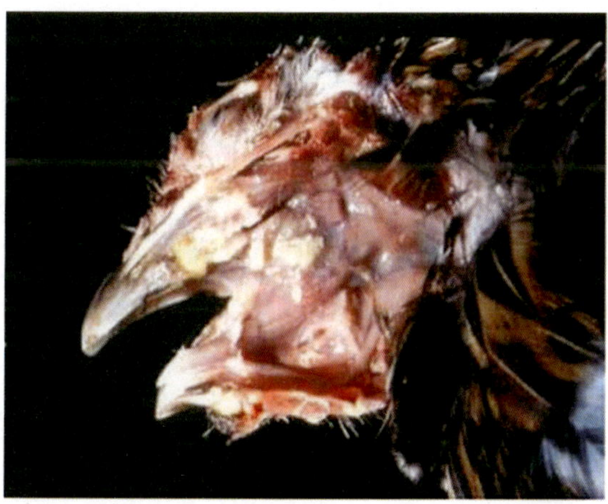

Fig. 41: Fowl pox; Diphtheritic lesions in the mouth cavity

Prevention and Control

1) Vaccination is the only suitable method for prevention and control. Maternal antibodies are of no value in the prevention of pox infection.
2) Vaccination of susceptible chickens with either pigeon pox or fowl pox vaccine is possible before exposure. Both vaccines contain live virus.

• Fowl pox vaccine

1) It is used in chickens and turkeys. Pigeons are not vaccinated with this vaccine.
2) In high-risk areas, chickens are vaccinated by wing web method at 4-6 weeks of age and revaccinated at 16-18 weeks of age; otherwise, one vaccination at 13-16 weeks of age is sufficient.
3) Turkeys are vaccinated by stick method in the thigh at 10-14 weeks of age and revaccinated before the start of laying. It is better to vaccinate every 3-4 months.

• Pigeon pox vaccine

1) Used in pigeons for regular vaccination and chickens and turkeys for primary vaccination.
2) Usually, pigeons are vaccinated by wing web method and chickens and turkeys by brush to denuded feather follicles. Can be used in chickens and turkeys of any age. Revaccination in chickens and turkeys is by fowl pox vaccine.
3) N.B. Vaccination produces a small lesion ("take") at the site of vaccination. A large percent of vaccinated birds should have "takes" about 7-10 days post-vaccination otherwise revaccination is necessary.

Treatment

There is no satisfactory treatment for pox.

38

Infectious Bursal Disease (IBD; Gumboro Disease)

IBD is an acute, contagious, viral disease of young chickens characterized by diarrhoea, vent pecking, trembling, incoordination, inflammation followed by atrophy of the bursa of Fabricius (BF) and by a variable degree of immunosuppression.

In the USA the disease was reported in Gumboro, Delaware in 1962, hence the name. The occurrence is worldwide.

Occurrence

Chickens - in other species, e.g. turkeys, not usually a problem. 1-10 weeks (usually 3-7 weeks) old birds are more susceptible.

Etiology

1) IBD virus (IBDV); an RNA virus belonging to the Birnaviridae family.
2) Serotypes of IBDV exist, designated as serotype 1 pathogenic and serotype 2 (less pathogenic or non-virulent). These can be differentiated by virus neutralization test but not by FAT and ELISA tests.

Transmission

The virus is shed in faeces and infection spreads horizontally through contaminated feed and water.

Clinical Signs

1) Mostly seen clinically between 3 and seven weeks.
2) Chicken under three weeks do not show clinical signs but exhibit severe immunosuppression, important for immunization program.
3) Classical IBD has a sudden onset, high morbidity reaching to 100%, spiking mortality (1-30%) and rapid recovery.

4) There may be tremor or unsteadiness, depression, anorexia, ruffled feathers, a droopy appearance and vent pecking.

5) Severe watery diarrhoea and dehydration (Figure 42).

6) The important aspect of this infection is the sub-clinical immunosuppressive effect, which may facilitate incidence of other diseases.

Gross Lesions

1) Birds are dehydrated in later stages.

2) Darkened discolouration of pectoral muscles.

3) Haemorrhages in the thigh and pectoral muscles (Figure 43).

4) Increased mucus in the intestine.

5) Bursa of Fabricius (BF)

   a) Day 2-3 PI gelatinous yellowish transudate; BF —> cream in colour (Figure 44).

   b) Day 3 PI increase in size and weight; BF —> dark red in color

   c) Day 4 PI BF double its normal weight

   d) Day 5 PI BF returns to normal weight and starts atrophy; BF —> gray

   e) Day 8 PI BF 1/3 its original weight, necrosis develops and lumen of BF is filled with caseous exudate.

6) Necrotic foci, petechiae or ecchymoses in the BF; sometimes extensive haemorrhage (Figure 45). Microscopically there is necrosis in bursal follicles (Figure 46).

7) Spleen; slightly enlarged and has small grey foci dispersed on the capsular surface.

8) Haemorrhages in the mucosa at the juncture of the proventriculus and gizzard.

9) Renal changes; kidneys may be swollen, and ureters may contain urates.

Diagnosis

1) Clinically, rapid onset, high morbidity, spiking mortality curve, and rapid recovery (5-7 days) from clinical signs.

2) Necropsy: characteristic gross changes and microscopic lesions in bursa of Fabricius.

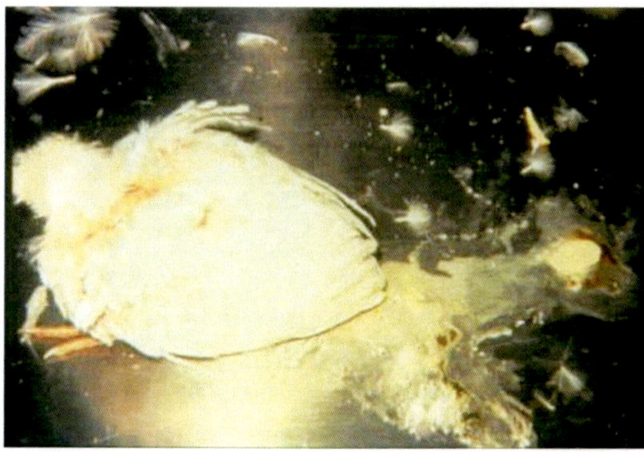

Fig. 42: IBD; Infected chicken is typically depressed showing ruffled feathers and watery diarrhea

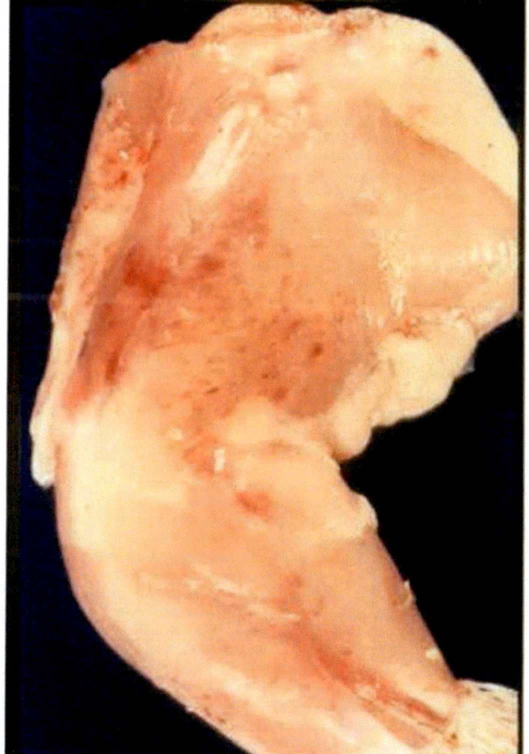

Fig. 43: IBD; Hemorrhages into the thigh muscles

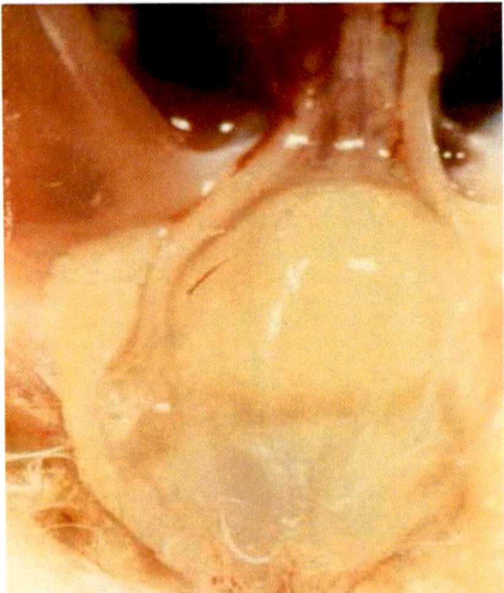

Fig. 44: IBD; Swollen and edematous bursa, 2-3 day PI

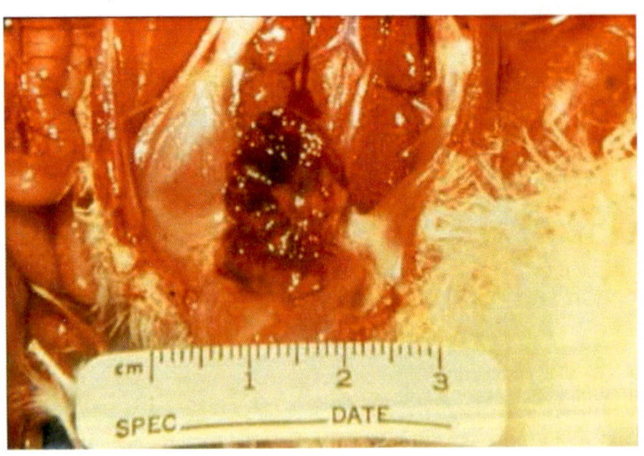

Fig.45: IBD; In some outbreaks bursa exhibits extensive hemorrhages in the lumen,

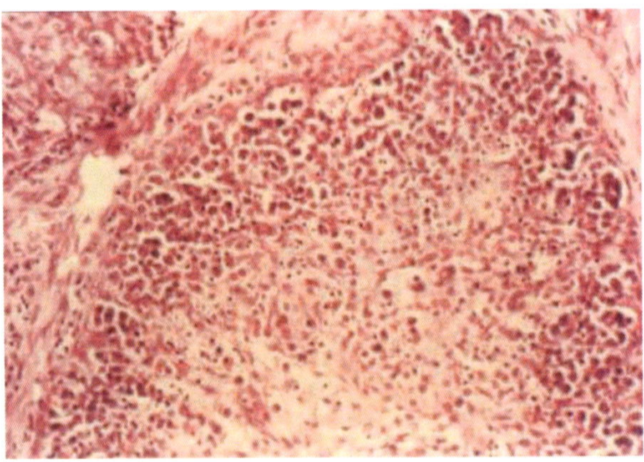

Fig. 46: IBD; Necrosis of the bursal follicles

3) Isolation and identification of the virus.

4) Serology: agar gel precipitation test, virus neutralization test, ELISA tests.

5) PCR based molecular techniques.

Prevention and Control

1) **Vaccination is the primary method for the control of IBD. Four types of vaccine are available.**

   a) **Live virus vaccines from virulent strains:** It is not usually used in chicks. It could be given to breeders at 10-14 weeks of age for booster vaccination.

   b) **Live virus vaccines from intermediate strains:** Usually used for chicks having maternal antibodies.

   c) **Live virus vaccine from attenuated strains:** It can be given to chicks with maternal antibodies, but it produces immunity if given by injection.

   d) **Oil emulsion killed virus vaccine:** Usually used in breeder birds for booster immunization.

1) Immunization of Chicks

The age for vaccination is decided depending on the level of maternal antibodies which normally protects chicks for 1-3 weeks. Chicks having a high level of maternal immunity may be vaccinated at 2-3 weeks of age in drinking water with a vaccine made of intermediate strain (TAD Gumboro/D78).

Chicks without maternal antibodies can be vaccinated at one day of age, and repeated at 21- 28 day of age.

2) Immunization of Breeder Birds

The first vaccination is done as for chicks. Second vaccination could be repeated after three weeks in endemic areas. A booster vaccination is done by injection of killed virus vaccine at 16-18 weeks of age.

39

Marek's Disease

Marek's disease is a herpesvirus-induced neoplastic disease of chickens characterized by infiltration of various nerve trunks and/or organs with pleomorphic lymphoid cells. Marek's disease is world wide in distribution. Marek's Disease has been named after Josef Marek who published the disease in 4 roosters in 1907.

Occurrence

In chickens only, however turkeys and quail have limited susceptibility. Lesions similar to MD have been seen in pheasants, ducks, pigeons, geese, canaries, budgerigars, swans and great horned owls. However, aetiology for lesions in these species has not been proved. It may appear at 3-4 weeks but usually after eight weeks, with major losses from 12-25 weeks. Morbidity and mortality varies depending on the virulence of MDV.

Etiology

1) Herpes virus (MDV) which belongs to herpes group B, a cell associated herpes virus.
2) On the basis of serotyping, MDV has been classified into three serotypes:
   a) Serotype I : Virulent and less virulent strains
   b) Serotype II: Nonvirulent strains
   c) Serotype III : Turkey herpes virus (HVT) strain; non pathogenic but antigenically related to MDV.
   - Based on virulence associated with Serotype I, four groups of MDV are recognized: mMDV (mild virulence); vMDV (virulent); vvMDV (very virulent) and vv+ MDV (very very virulent).
3) There is cross- reaction between serotypes.
4) New strains of high virulence are appearing in various countries.

Clinical Signs

1) These are usually associated with the involvement of nerves and tissues including visceral organs. Since one or several nerves of the body may be affected, the clinical signs associated with nerve lesions vary from one bird to another.

Clinical signs connected with the lesion in major nerves of the body are as under.

	Affected Nerves	Clinical Signs
(i)	Brachial nerves	Paralysis of wings
(ii)	Sciatic nerves	Paralysis of legs, usually one leg is stretched forward and another backward.
(iii)	Cervical spinal nerves	Torticollis of neck.
(iv)	Vagus nerves	Impaction of crop & respiratory signs.
(v)	Intercostal nerves	Respiratory distress
(vi)	Celiac or mesenteric nerves	Diarrhea and emaciation

There may be temporary recovery in paralytic signs in few birds, but the clinical signs reappear again.

2) In a few birds blindness develops as a result of the involvement of iris of the eyes. Pupil at first, is seen irregular and later become small as pinpoint opening (Figure 47).

3) In some acute outbreaks, no Specific paralytic signs are seen, and majority of birds die with out clinical signs.

4) In a proportion of birds, non-specific clinical signs - like loss of weight, anorexia, diarrhoea, dehydration and paleness are observed. These develop in birds, which are unable to reach to feed and water.

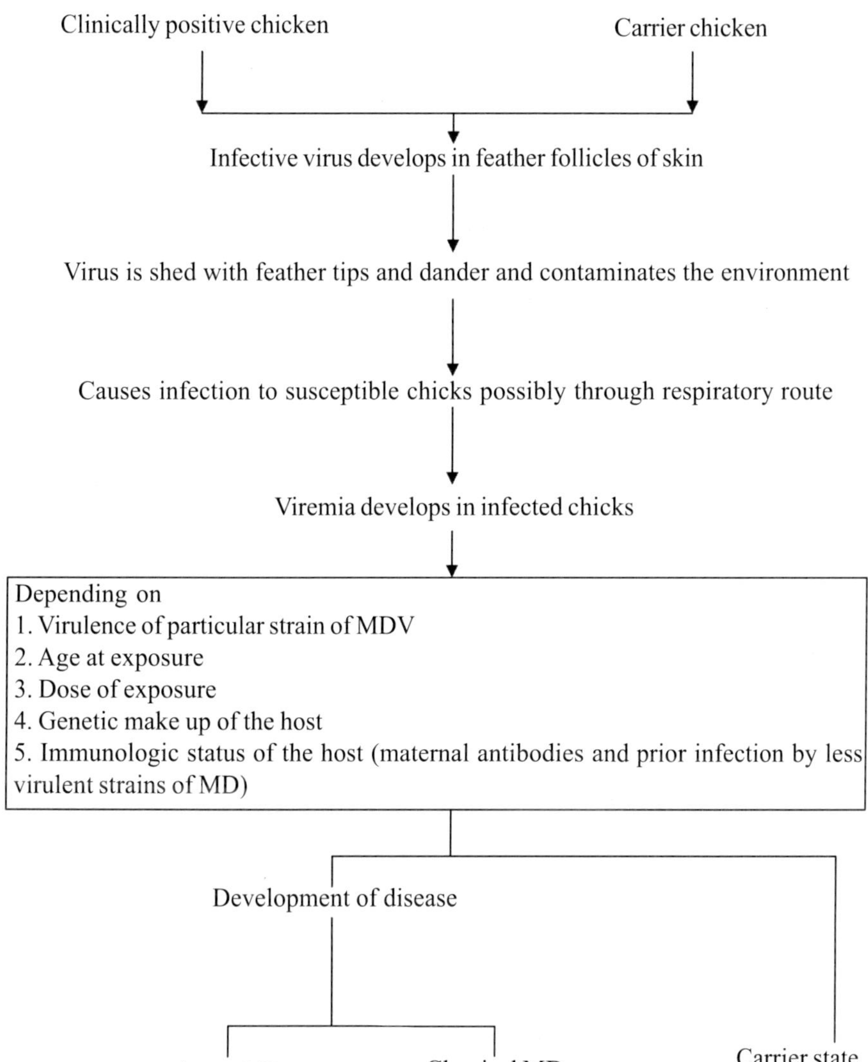

Lesions

• Gross Lesions

1) In Central Nervous System (CNS)

Brain and spinal cord do not show gross lesions.

2) Nerves

Nerves show loss of cross striations, become grey or yellow in colour losing its normal shining. There is localised or diffuse enlargement of the affected portion of the nerve. The enlargement may be 2-3 times than normal size. The involvement of the nerve may be unilateral or bilateral (Figure 48).

3) Visceral lesions are seen in the form of lymphoid tumours which are difficult to differentiate from lymphoid leukosis. However, grossly the visceral tumours are more common in the acute form of MD.

4) Lesions may be in lung, liver, heart, kidney, intestine, mesentery, spleen, adrenal, pancreas, proventriculus, iris, muscles (Figure 49) and skin (Figure 50) but the lesions in gonads are more often seen.

Histopathology

Brain and spinal cord: Perivascular cuffing with small lymphocytes. Also small area of cellular infiltration with pleomorphic mononuclear cells are found in spinal cord and ganglia.

Microscopic lesions in the skin include infiltration of pleomorphic lymphoid cells around the hair follicles and below the epidermis (Figure 51).

Visceral tumors and nerves show infiltration of pleomorphic cells, which are made up of various stages of lymphocytes and plasma cells (Figure 52).

Diagnosis

1) Symptoms of paralysis and postmortem lesions (location of the neoplastic lesions) usually are enough for a tentative diagnosis. Paralysis is often unilateral affecting leg or wing.

2) Nerve involvement (when present), absence of bursal lesions, and pleomorphi lymphocytes comprising lesions.

3) Virus isolation.

4) **Serology:** Demonstration of antibody can be done by FAT, AGPT, serum neutralization test and ELISA.

5) Detection of antigen: Antigen can be detected in tissues (most suitable skin) of chicken by fluorescent antibody test (FAT) and Immunodiffusion test (AGPT).

6) PCR assays.

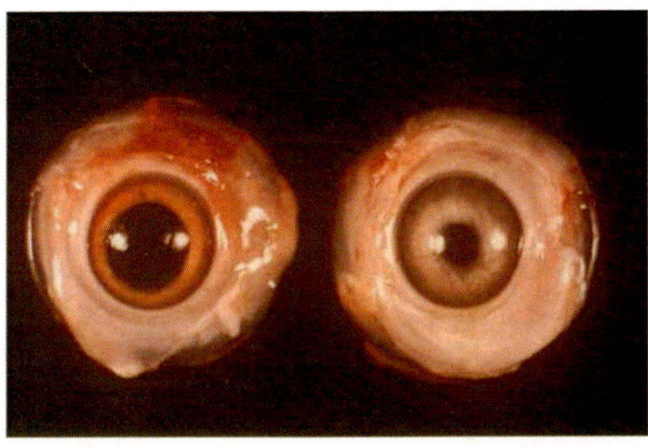

Fig. 47: MD. Eye lesions-Cellular infiltration in iris (right) causing white discoloration. Pupil is irregular and does not respond to light intensity

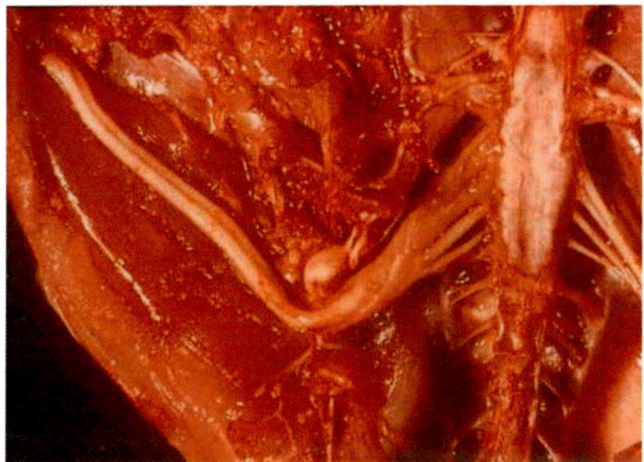

Fig. 48: MD. Involved sciatic nerve is thickened, dull and yellowish in contrast to glistening white unaffected right nerve

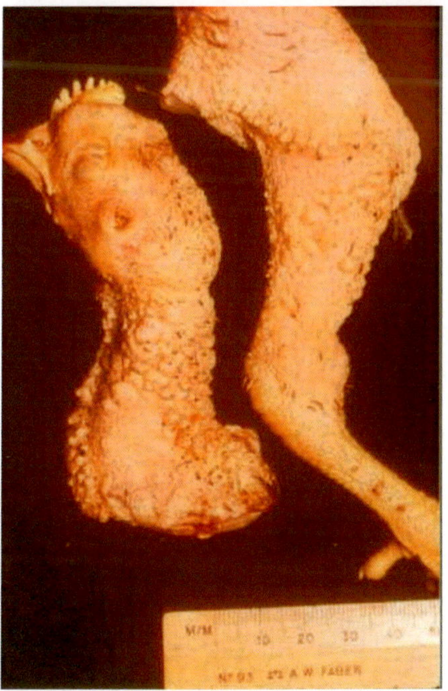

Fig. 49: MD. Tumors marked on the skin,

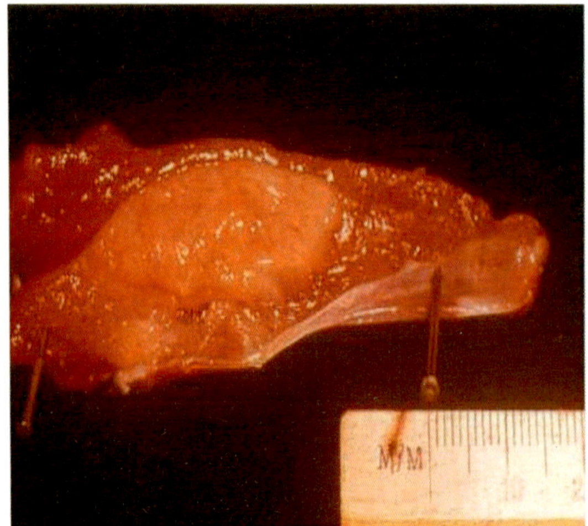

Fig. 50: MD. Tumor in the muscle

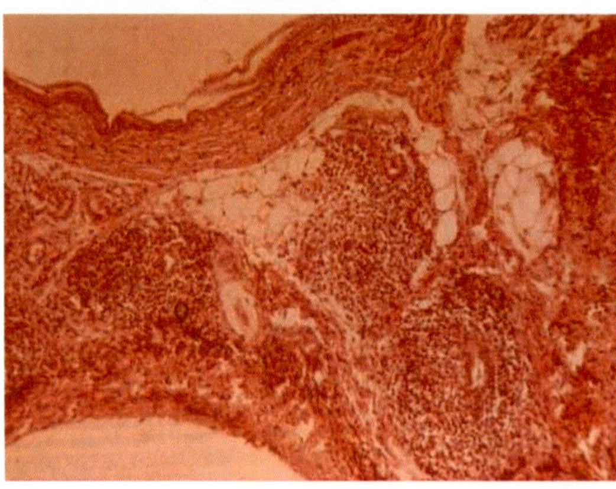

Fig.51: MD. Microscopic lesions in the skin, infiltration of pleomorphic lymphoid cells around the hair follicles and below the epidermis,

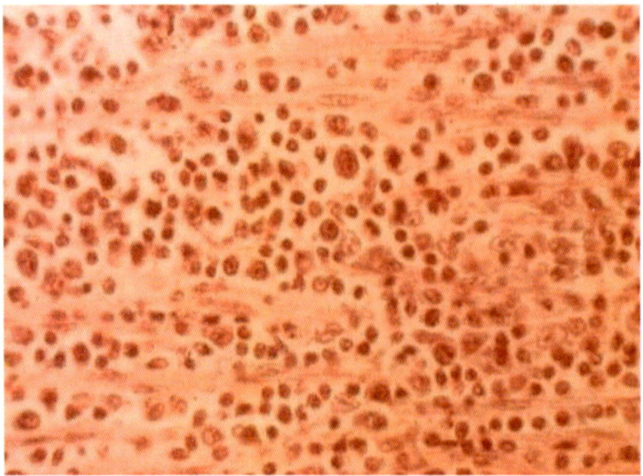

Fig.52: MD. Microscopic lesions- pleomorphic lymphoid cells infiltration

Differential Diagnosis

Lymphoid leukosis, reticuloendotheliosis, myeloblastosis, erythroblastosis, carcinoma of the ovary, other neoplasms, riboflavin deficiency, tuberculosis, histomoniasis, genetic grey eye, Newcastle disease, avian encephalomyelitis, perosis, and joint infections or injuries.

Prevention and Control

1) Vaccination. Commercial vaccines are available, produced from any of the three serotypes of viruses.

    a) Attenuated serotype 1 MDV

    b) Naturally avirulent serotype 2 MDV

    c) Turkey Herpes virus (HVT) which has been used most because it is cheap to produce and the cell-free virus of HVT can be lyophilized.

    - Vaccination is done at one day of age preferably in the hatchery by intramuscular injection. The dose of the vaccine is usually 1 ml containing more than 1000 P.F.U. Now in ovo-vaccination is being practised by hatcheries. Protection from the vaccine is usually 80-100%, and the protection is usually life long. Vaccinated chicks are susceptible to infection with virulent MDV, but lymphoma is not formed.

2) Vaccination of day old chicks at hatchery and avoidance of infection during immediate. Post-Vaccination period (7-10 days). This requires careful sanitation and disinfection since MDV survives well for months in poultry houses.

Treatment

There is no effective treatment for MD. Birds with tumours or multiple skin lesions are condemned at slaughter.

SECTION-2
Bacterial Diseases

40

Avian Leukosis (LL)

(Lymphoid Leukosis, LL)

LL is a retrovirus-causes, neoplastic disease of semi-mature or mature chickens characterized by a gradual onset in a flock, persistent low mortality and neoplasia of, the bursa of Fabricius (BF) with metastasis to many other internal organs especially the liver, spleen and kidney.

Etiology

Caused by viruses of leukosis/sarcoma group. The viruses of this group are divided into six subgroups namely A, B, C, D, E and J. There are various antigenic types within subgroups. Viruses within subgroups cross-neutralize. Thus, the strains of avian leukosis/sarcoma group are classified according to main lesions they produce and the subgroup envelope they have. Subgroup A and B cause lymphoid leukosis; subgroup C and D are rare, and subgroup E is not pathogenic for poultry.

Leukosis/sarcoma virus (a family of retroviruses known as avian leukosis viruses). Usually, Subgroup A and B principally cause lymphoid leukosis.

Predisposing Factors

Genetic susceptibility.

Transmission

Transmission cycle of leukosis/sarcoma virus

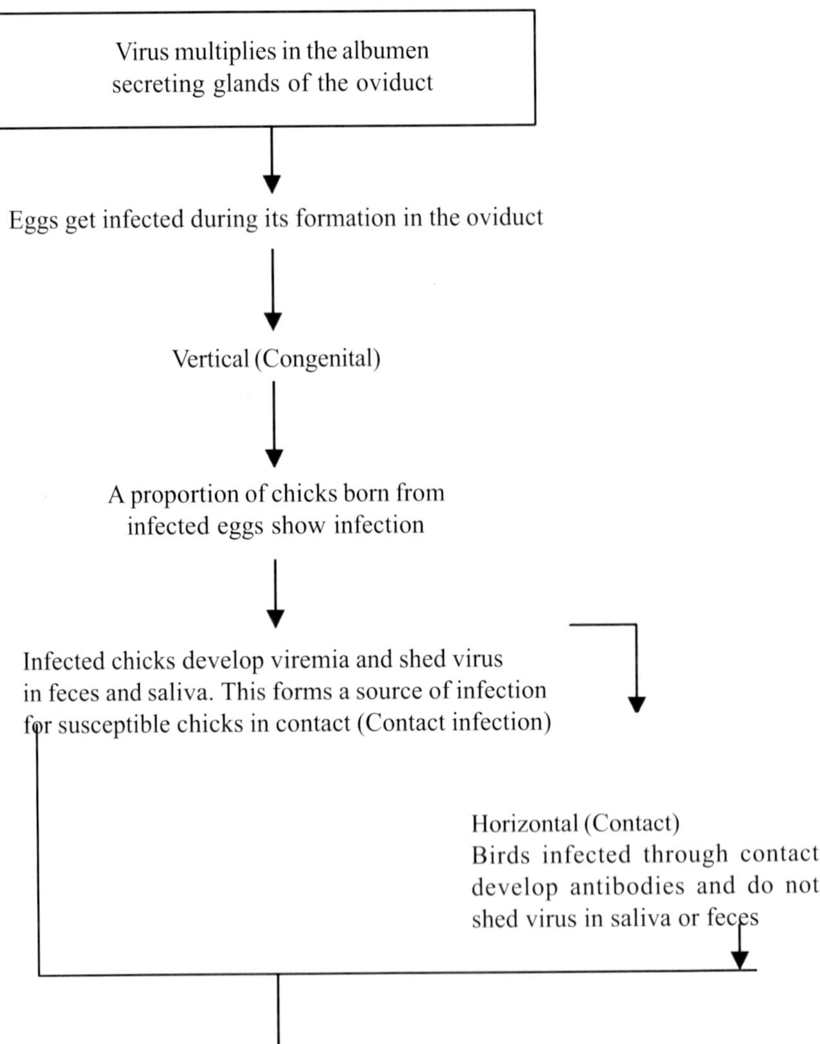

On maturity these birds become shedders of virus in eggs

Clinical Signs

1) There are no specific clinical signs. Symptoms otherwise are variable depending on which organ affected.
2) The course of the disease is prolonged, but once the clinical signs begin to develop, the course is quite rapid.

3) Paralysis is not a feature.
4) There is a loss of appetite and birds become weak with unthriftiness or emaciation.
5) Anemia develops seen as pale head parts (comb, mucous membranes).
6) Abdominal enlargement is resulting from massive hepatomegaly and can be detected by palpation or by insertion of a finger into the cloaca to detect the enlarged BF.
7) Mortality varies from 5-15%.

Lesions Gross

1) Lymphoid leukosis - a common manifestation is 'big liver disease' - other forms are erythroblastosis, myeloblastosis, nephroma, hemangiomas, etc.
2) Lymphomas are seen in many organs in chickens at 16 weeks of age or older especially in the liver, kidney (Figure 53), ovary and BF. Tumors may also develop in other organs as well, such as kidney, lung, gonad, heart, bone marrow and mesentery. The size of a tumour and number of organs affected are variable.

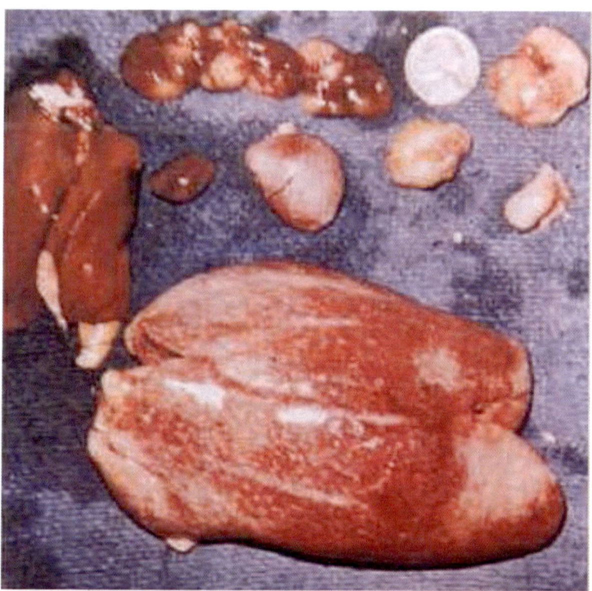

Fig. 53: Lymphoid leucosis: Grayish solid tumors in the kidney, liver and spleen. Typically affected organ: enlarged, pinkish liver(lower organ), contrasted with normal liver(upper left), dark brown, tumorous kidneys (top) are common, as is the enlarged spleen, contrasted with normal spleen on its left.

3) Tumors may have following morphology:

   a) Nodular: spherical or flattened tumours may be present close to the surface of the organ. Size varies from 0.5 mm to 5.0 cm.

   b) Miliary: Small nodules less than 2 mm in diameter but uniformly distributed throughout the parenchyma of the affected organ.

   c) Diffuse: The growth of a tumour is diffuse, and the organ is uniformly enlarged, and friable. The colour of the affected organ becomes slightly greyish.

4) The tumours particularly in the nodular, form are soft, smooth and glistening. The cut surface is greyish to creamy white but without any area of necrosis.

5) Anemic birds have pale blood, which is usually slow to clot.

6) Incision of the BF may reveal small nodular lesions not otherwise obvious.

Histopathology

Neoplastic cells in tumours are uniformly lymphoblastic. Proliferating tumour cells displace and compress the cells of the organ, rather than infiltrating between them.

Comparison of epizootiologic and pathologic features of Marek's disease (MD) and Lymphoid Leukosis (LL)

Characteristic	MD	LL
Age of occurrence:		
Peak time	2-7 months	4-10 months
Clinical signs:		
Paralysis	Common (+++)	Absent (-)
Gross lesions:		
Liver	Common (+++)	Common (+++)
Spleen	Common (+++)	Common (+++)
Nerves	Common (+++)	Absent (-)
Skin	Common (+++)	Rare (+)
Bursa tumor	Rare (+)	Common (+++)
Bursa atrophy	Common (+++)	Rare (+)
Gonads	Common (+++)	Rare (+)
Heart	Common (+++)	Rare (+)
Intestine	Rare (+)	Common (+++)
Lungs	Common (+++)	Rare (+)
Kidney	Common (+++)	Common (+++)
Microscopic lesions:		
Pleomorphic cells	Yes / (+)	No / (-)
Uniform blast cells	No / (-)	Yes / (+)
Bursa of Fabricius tumor	Interfollicular	Intrafollicular
Surface antigens:		
MATSA	+ (5-40%)	- (Absent)
IgM	+ (<5%)	+++ (91-99%)
B-cell	+ (3-25%)	+++ (91-99%)
T-cell	+++ (60-90%)	+ (Rare)

Prevention and Control

Control by breaking the transmission cycle of virus from parents to chicks. Vaccination has been attempted, but still, there is no suitable vaccine for leukosis.

41

Myelocytomatosis

The neoplastic disease primarily of broiler breeders and broilers causing serious economic losses in the commercial poultry industry. A case has been recorded in a budgerigar.

Etiology

ALV-J subgroup, identified in 1988. It became widespread in commercial meat type poultry in the 1990's. Transmission of ALV-J is much higher than other subgroups thus making control much more difficult.

Lesions

Tumors are distinctive dull, yellow-white, soft and friable and diffuse or nodular.

Histology

Histologically tumours consist of compact masses of uniform myelocytes with very little stroma (Figure 54). Tumor nodules made of immature granulocytes are found in liver, spleen, kidney, sternum and other tissues. Hemangiosarcoma, histiocytoma, myxoma, carcinoma in the liver, fibrosarcoma, lymphoma, ganglioneuroma and renal tumours have also been associated with sub group J virus.

Diagnosis

1) Clinical signs and lesions: (tumours) in young birds
2) Virus isolation
3) Serology – ELISA
4) PCR- PCR in feather pulp.

   Positive result in 90% infected embryos.

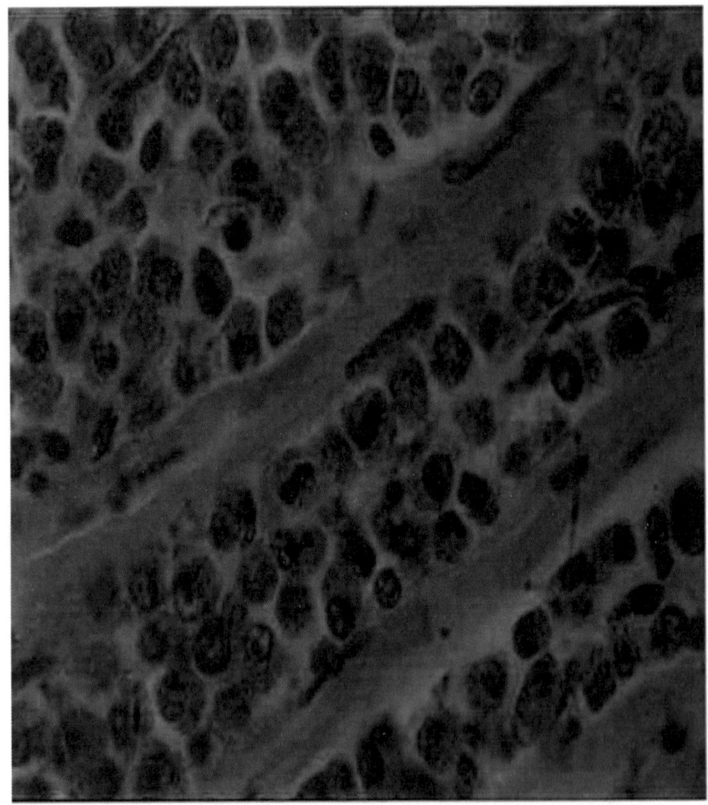

Fig. 54: Myelocytomatosis: Infiltration of myeloid cells

42

Reticuloendotheliosis

Term endotheliosis designates a variety of syndrome caused by a reticuloendothelial virus (REV). REV caused syndromes have been demonstrated world wide.

Etiology

Based on replication of the virus in chicken fibroblast cell culture, two strains are known: replication defective T strain and the non-defective A strain. The REV manifests three distinct diseases syndromes:

1) A runting disease syndrome; caused by A strain
2) Chronic neoplasia of lymphoid and other tissues; caused by A strain
3) Acute reticulum cell neoplasia; caused by T strain

Host

Common in chicken, turkey, ducks and many other species of birds.

Transmission

The virus is transmitted horizontally by physical contact with infected birds. The virus is excreted in faeces. Mosquitoes and other insects may transmit the virus as passive carriers. Low-grade transmission through the egg has also been demonstrated.

Clinical Signs

In runting syndrome birds are pale, anaemic and stunted with feather abnormalities. Mortality is low but culling rate is very high, the cause of significant economic loss. Depression and death are the only clinical signs in birds with chronic lymphomas. Clinical signs with acute reticulum cell neoplasia are rarely observed because of rapid high mortality.

Lesions

1) In runting syndrome, main injuries are atrophy of thymus and bursa of Fabricius. In some birds enlargement of nerves, anaemia and inflammatory lesions in the intestine and proventriculus may be found. Bird suffer from secondary infections because of immunosuppression in REV.
2) In chronic lymphoma, syndrome lesions resemble Mareks' disease with involvement of nerves, and tumours in liver, heart and thymus. Tumors appear as early as six weeks of age.
3) In acute reticulum cell neoplasia, There is hepatomegaly and splenomegaly with diffuse infiltration of cells of the reticuloendothelial system. Similar lesions may also be present in heart, kidney, gonads and pancreas.

Diagnosis

1) In addition to clinical signs and lesions, demonstration of REV in lesions is of great diagnostic value.
2) Serology performed by FAT, VN test, Agar gel precipitation test, and ELISA is a reliable method for the diagnosis of REV.
3) Identification of REV through PCR technique is valuable in diagnosis.

Differential Diagnosis

Tumors of REV be differentiated with that of tumours produced in Marek's disease and lymphoid leucosis. Runting syndrome is differentiated from other immunosuppressive conditions and malnutrition.

Treatment, prevention and Control

There is no treatment for REV infection. Because of no effective vaccine, biosecurity including insect control is advisable in the prevention of the REV infection.

43

Avian Nephritis

Etiology

Avian Nephritis Virus (ANV), an RNA virus is Astro virus under the genus Avastrovirus in Astroviridae family. Strains of ANV exist. ANV is very resistant and stable in the environment.

Host

Only young chickens. However, ANV has been detected in turkeys, ducks, guinea fowl and pigeons. Infection is reported in commercial chickens all over the world.

Transmission

ANV is transmitted horizontally by direct or indirect contact, through faecal oral route. Vertical transmission has been suggested through the egg based on field observations.

Clinical Signs

ANV affects young chicks and causes growth depression (runting syndrome). Susceptibility decreases with age.

Lesions

1) Nephritis with swollen kidneys, prominent ureters and visceral gout.
2) Histologically, there are necrosis and degeneration of epithelial cells of the proximal the convoluted tubules with interstitial infiltration of granulocytes and lymphocytes.

Diagnosis

1) In commercial flocks, ANV infection is highly prevalent but subclinical.
2) Demonstration of ANV antigen through IHC or FAT and antibodies through various serological tests are helpful in the diagnosis.

3) Isolation and identification of virus through RT-PCR and sequencing gives a confirmatory diagnosis.

Differential Diagnosis

Nephritis caused by certain strains of Infectious bronchitis virus (IBV) need be differentiated. In IBV in addition to kidney lesions, there are clinical signs and lesions in the respiratory system.

Treatment and Prevention

There is no specific treatment. No vaccine is available for ANV. Strict biosecurity including effective disinfection is practised for prevention.

44

Avian Influenza (AI; Influenza; Fowl Plague)

AI is a viral disease affecting the respiratory, enteric or nervous system of many kinds of birds. The most virulent form is an acute, generalized disease characterized in poultry by a short course and extremely high mortality.

Occurrence Species

Theoretically all avian species are susceptible, but in farming, turkeys are the primary targets. Migratory birds transmit strains of the virus internationally.

Etiology

An RNA orthomyxovirus; Type A Influenza virus: many strains exist. Strains of AI virus based on pathogenicity are classified :

1) HPAI (High pathogenic avian influenza virus- fowl plague like)
2) MPAI (mildly pathogenic avian influenza virus).

Epizootiology

1) Wild and domesticated waterfowl are the major reservoir of influenza viruses and may excrete virus for long periods. The virus has been recovered from water from lakes and ponds utilized by infected wild ducks.
2) Imported exotic birds are a potential threat to cage birds, wild birds or poultry.
3) Transmission from contaminated shoes, clothing, crates and other equipment occurs.

Clinical Signs

HPAI Viruses

1) In wild birds and domestic ducks, a few clinical signs are seen.
2) In chicken and turkey signs vary from sudden death to less fulminating disorders. Later in 3-7 days PI chicken and turkey, show nervous disorders exhibited as torticollis, opisthotonus and inability to stand.
3) The decline in feed and water consumption, lower egg production, mild respiratory signs as sneezing, coughing and rales may be seen.
4) Mortality and morbidity are very high, 50-90%.

MPAI Viruses

1) In wild birds, no clinical signs and no mortality are observed.
2) In domestic poultry (chicken and turkey) most frequent symptoms are respiratory exhibited by coughing, sneezing, rales, rattles and lacrimation.
3) Decreased feed and water consumption, lower egg production and occasional diarrhoea may be seen.
4) There is high morbidity and low mortality (<50%).

Lesions

HPAI Viruses

1) Edema, necrosis and haemorrhage in the skin and visceral organs.
2) In skin lesions of necrosis, haemorrhage and oedema are especially seen on the wattles and comb (Figure 55).
3) Hemorrhages are more marked on pericardium, pectoral muscles, proventriculus, gizzard and intestine.
4) Frequent necrosis and haemorrhage may be present in heart, lung, liver, kidney and brain.

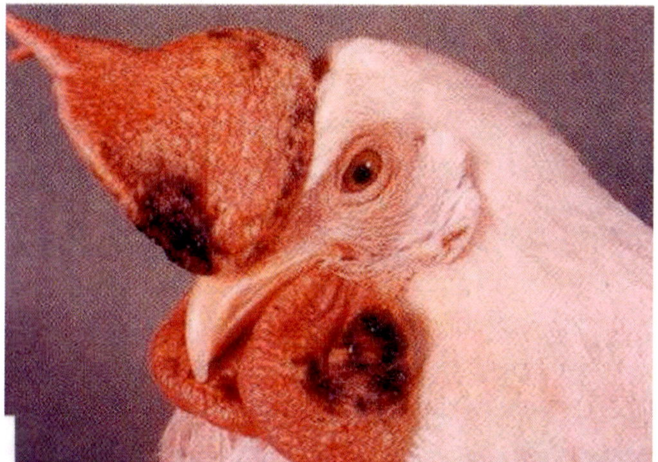

Fig.55: Avian Influenza. Multifocal necrosis and hemorrhage of comb and wattles

MPAI Viruses

1) Lesions are more in the respiratory tract seen as catarrhal/fibrinous, fibrinopurulent exudates in sinuses and trachea.
2) Catarrhal/ fibrinous exudates may be present in the peritoneal cavity.
3) Ovary and oviduct may show haemorrhages.

Diagnosis

1) Virus isolation is required in the initial stages of an outbreak.
2) Serology: HA, HI, ELISA and agar gel precipitation tests.
3) PCR based techniques for the confirmation of the diagnosis.
4) Specimens for diagnosis: tracheal and cloacal swabs of live or dead birds.

Differential Diagnosis

Newcastle disease and other paramyxovirus infections, infectious bronchitis, infectious laryngotracheitis, chlamydiosis, and mycoplasmosis.

Prevention and Control

AI is a Notifiable Disease

• Immediate Action

Confirmation of the diagnosis requires laboratory assessment of the virulence of the virus isolated. After the diagnosis of AI on the farm; **Quarantine** the farm and take the following action:

a) **With HPAI:** Inform appropriate authorities, who will put in place Government eradication procedure (quarantine, slaughter, disposal and clean up).

b) **With MPAI:** Prevent the spread of the disease beyond initial focus of outbreak; regulate the orderly and timely marketing of birds and eggs.

Long Term Action

1) Control is largely through prevention of exposure to influenza viruses.
2) Wild birds and waterfowl may introduce infection and should not be introduced into, or allowed direct or indirect contact with poultry flocks. Swine may also transmit the infection to domestic birds.
3) Quarantine controls on imports of domestic poultry or exotic birds.

Treatment

No specific medication.

Vaccination

Inactivated AI virus vaccines prevent clinical signs and mortality. However, protection is virus sub type specific. Vaccination may be useful after identification of virus type. Inactivated vaccines are recommended in the face of MPAI outbreaks. However, serological surveillance of such flocks is impeded as virus infection can occur and persist in the absence of the disease. Now vectored vaccines and DNA vaccines incorporating HA genes are in use. They protect a broad array of homologous HA sub type viruses. The advantage of such vaccines is in serological surveillance as vaccinated birds do not react to double diffusion test.

45

Avian Encephalomyelitis

(AE; Epidemic Tremor; Infectious Avian Encephalomyelitis)

AE is a viral infection of chickens, turkeys, pheasants and cortunix quail characterized in young birds by ataxia progressing to paralysis and, usually, by tremors of the head and neck. Infected adults usually show no signs. AE is world wide in distribution.

Occurrence Species

Chickens mainly affected – other species affected include turkey, pheasants, cortunix quail and pigeon.

Age Range

Chicks 1-3 weeks ('Tremor')

Adult layers (Lowered egg production)

Etiology

Infectious avian encephalomyelitis virus (AEV); belongs to genus Tremorvirus in Picornaviridae family. There are two pathotypes of AEV; one field strain-enterotrophic; another pathotype is embryo adapted strain. Serologically they are similar.

Transmission

1) During the acute phase of infection, layers infected with enterotrophic strain will shed virus in some of the eggs they lay; chicks from infected eggs may show signs of AEV at hatching or within a few days there from.
2) Enterotropic strain is present in the faeces of infected birds and will survive there for at least four weeks; thus virus may spread laterally to other chicks of the hatch.

3) Horizontal spread of the virus is important in large, mixed flocks.

4) Embryo adopted strain cause severe neurological signs when inoculated intracerebrally or parental routes. They do not spread horizontally.

Clinical Signs

Chicks

1) In natural outbreak depression, ataxia progressing to paralysis and prostration, and fine muscular tremors of the head and neck followed by death are seen in 1-2 weeks of age. Tremors are more pronounced when chicks are disturbed or excited. Tremors may continue for a variable period, and the reoccur irregularly.

2) Morbidity may reach 60%.

3) Survivors fail to thrive and may develop cataracts and impaired vision.

Adults

No clinical signs but a slight drop in egg production (5%- 10%) is possible.

Lesions

- **Gross**

Usually, there are no gross lesions

Histopathology

1) CNS lesions of disseminated nonsuppurative encephalomyelitis with widespread and marked perivascular cuffing in the brain and spinal cord.

2) Swelling and chromatolysis of neurons in nuclei (nucleus rotundus and nucleus ovoidalis) in the midbrain and cerebellum.

3) Dense lymphoid aggregates in the muscle of the proventriculus and gizzard.

Diagnosis / Sampling

1) History, the age of birds, clinical signs, and histopathology of CNS gives a strong presumptive diagnosis.

2) Virus isolation and identification using susceptible embryos may be required to confirm the diagnosis. PCR based techniques are used in identification.

3) Serological tests using, ELISA, Neutralization and immunodiffusion may be helpful. FAT on CNS to detect antigen will be confirmatory.

4) Rising antibody titers in layers following a slump in egg production is suggestive of infection with AEV.

5) Differentiation from other diseases causing signs of CNS disease in young birds: ND, MD, arboviral infection, vitamin deficiencies (E, A, and riboflavin), mycotic encephalitis, brain abscesses, toxicities (salt, pesticides, etc.).

Specimens required for Diagnosis

1) Live sick chicks

2) Brain, spinal cord, pancreas, liver, proventriculus and heart in 10% formalin and 50% glycerine separately

3) Serum

Prevention and Control

- **Immediate Action**

  a) Kill affected chicks

  b) Long Term

Protection results from vaccination of young breeders with live vaccine in drinking water at 14-16 weeks of age. Vaccination prevents vertical transmission through egg borne route and maternal antibodies protect progeny during the first 2-3 weeks, the critical time of infection.

Treatment

No treatment is available.

46

Coronaviral Enteritis of Turkeys (CVE)

(Blue comb disease, mud fever, transmissible enteritis, infectious enteritis)

Etiology

A turkey coronavirus (TCV).

Hosts

Turkeys of all ages, but the disease is mostly observed in young turkeys (first few weeks old).

Transmission

The virus is shed in faeces in infected turkeys. Recovered birds shed virus in faeces for several months. The infection is by contact of susceptible birds with infected birds or their faeces. TCV spread from farm to farm by personnel, equipment and vehicles.

Clinical Signs

In young poults and growing turkeys, the onset is sudden, 1-5 days after infection. Birds go off feed and water and are depressed. They lose weight and have watery, frothy diarrhoea. A few birds show darkening of skin and the head. Morbidity may reach 100%, but mortality varies from 5 to 50% In adult turkeys, the clinical signs are similar to those seen in poults but are less marked. However, there is drop in egg production, and some eggs shells are chalky. The course of the disease is usually two weeks. Recovery leaves flock with an uneven size of birds.

Lesions

Lesions are principally in the intestinal tract and cloacal bursa. Intestinal contents, especially in ceca, are watery and gaseous. The duodenum is swollen and pale. Petechial haemorrhages may be present on the mucosa of the intestine. The pancreas may have numerous white chalky spots. Ureters and kidneys may contain urates. Cloacal bursa may show atrophy

Diagnosis

1) Typical clinical signs and gross lesions are suggestive of TCV.
2) Filtered intestinal contents and bursa of Fabricius can be inoculated into 1-4 day- old turkey poults for infectivity test and into developing turkey embryos (>15 days) for virus isolation.
3) FA test is used on tissue sections from embryos and intestine of infected turkeys.
4) ELISA is another sensitive method to diagnose TCV.
5) Virus neutralization test is also of choice in the diagnosis of TCV.
6) PCR and EM may also be used in the diagnosis.

Treatment

No effective treatment is known. However, antibiotics and other drugs reduce mortality by controlling secondary infections.

Control

Since virus remains viable for a longer period on premises, thorough cleaning and disinfection of premises after complete depopulation is the best method of control.

No vaccine is available.

47

Hemorrhagic Enteritis of Turkeys

(HE; BLOODY GUT)

It is an acute disease of turkeys, occurring in 6-7 wk. -Old turkeys, but has been seen in younger and older turkeys as well. The disease is worldwide in distribution.

Etiological Agent

It belongs to adenovirus type II. A serologically indistinguishable virus from HE virus, causes marble spleen disease (MSD) in confinement reared pheasants (3-8 months old). The disease shows predominantly respiratory signs. A virus of the same group causes avian adenovirus group II splenomegaly (AAS) in chickens.

Natural Hosts

Turkey, pheasants, Chicken, guinea fowls and psittacines. Experimental infection in golden pheasants, bobwhite quail, peafowl and chukars has been produced without the death of the host.

Transmission

The epizootiology of HE is not well known. **Unlike other adenoviruses, it is not transmitted through an egg.** It is probably transmitted through fomites. Once introduced in turkey flock, it is spread through ingestion of contaminated faeces. Infection is known to reoccur in infected farms.

Clinical Signs

1) Sudden death is often the initial sign.
2) Birds become depressed with the drop in feed and water consumption. Droppings contain blood. Blood may be seen oozing from the vent or sticking on feathers around the vent.
3) The course of the disease is usually 6-10 days with an average mortality of 5-10%. Occasionally mortality may be as high as 60%.

4) Pheasants with MSD and chickens with AAS show depression, weakness, dyspnea and asphyxia.

Lesions

1) Birds are in the good flesh but appear pale because of blood loss.
2) The small intestine is distended, is dark red to black and filled with reddish brown bloody contents. The intestinal mucosa is congested, and occasional turkeys show fibrinous enteritis.
3) Spleens are enlarged, friable and mottled.
4) The liver is enlarged, hemorrhagic. Petechial haemorrhages are found on other visceral organs including subcutaneous tissue, breast and thigh muscles.
5) Pheasants with MSD and chickens with AAS show enlarged mottled spleen. Lungs are congested and edematous; possible cause of acute death.

Diagnosis

1) Typical history and gross lesions are suggestive of diagnosis for HE.
2) Demonstration of intranuclear inclusions in RE cells of spleen and small intestine.
3) Virus isolation and identification: Does not grow in embryos. Six weeks old turkeys are inoculated per os with splenic pulp (suspected tissue). Lesions of HE develop in 5-6 days.

Serology

AGP is used. ELISA, PCR and IFA and Immunoperoxidase methods can also be of use.

Treatment

S/C injection (0.5-1.0 ml) of immune antiserum from recovered turkeys. Antibiotics to prevent secondary coli septicemia.

Control

Live tissue culture vaccine in drinking water given at 4-6 weeks of age prevents HE.

Strict biosecurity measures prevent the infection.

48

Duck Virus Enteritis (DVE, Duck Plague)

Etiology

Herpes Virus

Variation in pathogenicity of virus strains has been reported, but all strains appear identical immunologically.

Occurrence

The disease was first reported in the Netherlands in 1923. The disease has been confirmed in France, Belgium, Canada, India, Thailand, England, Hungary, Austria, Denmark and Vietnam, and suspected in China.

Hosts

It is the disease of ducks, geese and swans.

Transmission

Direct contact between infected and susceptible birds.

Indirectly by contact with a, contaminated environment especially water.

Clinical Signs

1) All age birds ranging from 7-day old ducklings to mature breeder flocks are susceptible. Clinical signs appear in 3-7 days after exposure and mortality follow in 2-5 days. Mortality varies from 5 to 100%.

2) High sudden mortality is often the first observation. Most birds die in good flesh. As the disease progresses, more signs follow.

These include weakness, ataxia, photophobia, nasal and eye discharge, extreme thirst and watery diarrhoea with soiled vent. Many sick birds sit with drooping wings and head down. Majority of positive clinical birds die.

Lesions

DVE lesions are the sequel of vascular damage and degenerative changes in parenchymatous organs.

1) Petechial, ecchymotic or larger haemorrhages are found in the heart (Figure 56), visceral organs and serous membranes. On the heart, hemorrhages give the surface a red " paint brush" appearance.
2) Lesions in the digestive tract are present in the oral cavity, oesophagus (Figure 57), ceca, rectum and cloaca. Elevated, yellow, white crusty plaques later cover initial haemorrhages in these sites. There is haemorrhage and or necrosis in the annular bands or discs of lymphoid tissue along the intestine (Figure 58).
3) In the early stage, the liver is pale with pinpoint haemorrhage and necrotic foci (Figure 59). In later stages liver tissue turns dark bronze or bile stained, and has larger white areas of necrosis.
4) Microscopically, intranuclear inclusion bodies are identified in degenerating hepatocytes, epithelial cells of digestive system and lymphoid organs.

Diagnosis

1) Typical gross lesions and demonstration of intra-nuclear inclusions.
2) Confirmation is done by isolation and identification of the virus. Virus initially grows in duck embryos and not in chicken embryos. Virus neutralization test is used in identification.
3) IF tests can be used to detect viral antigens in cell cultures or tissue sections.

Differential Diagnosis

From duck virus hepatitis, pasteurellosis, necrotic enteritis and New castle disease.

Treatment

No effective treatment.

Prevention and Control

It is a noticeable disease in many countries. All outbreaks to be reported to appropriate authorities. Vaccination has been authorized in certain areas. A modified live virus vaccine has been used to prevent and control outbreaks in USA and Canada. It is given 0.5 ml S/C or I/M in ducklings over two wk. of age. Revaccination is done annually.

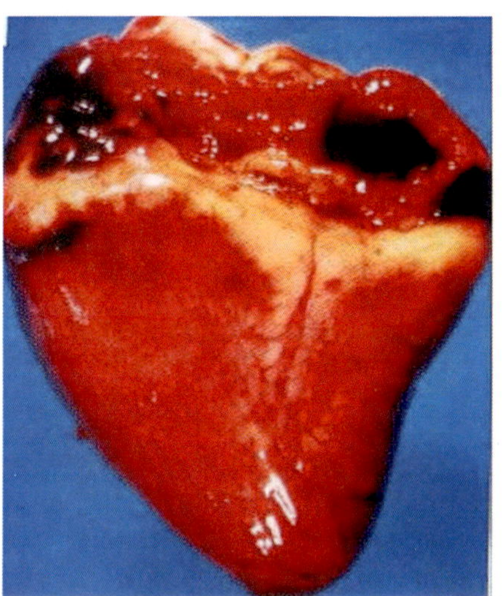

Fig. 56: DVE lesions; petechial hemorrhages on the epicardium

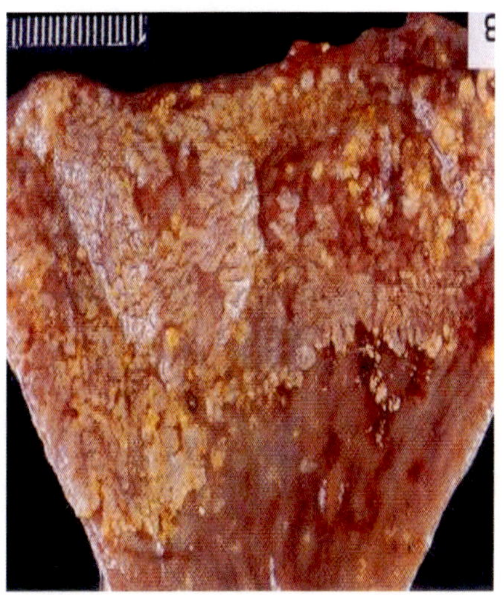

Fig. 57: DVE; extensive ulceration of esophageal mucosa

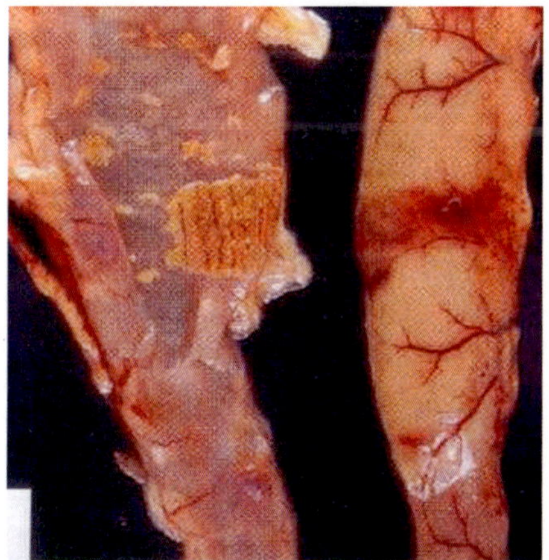

Fig. 58: DVE; band of red hemorrhagic areas on the serosal surface of the intestine, necrosis of GALT and ulceration,

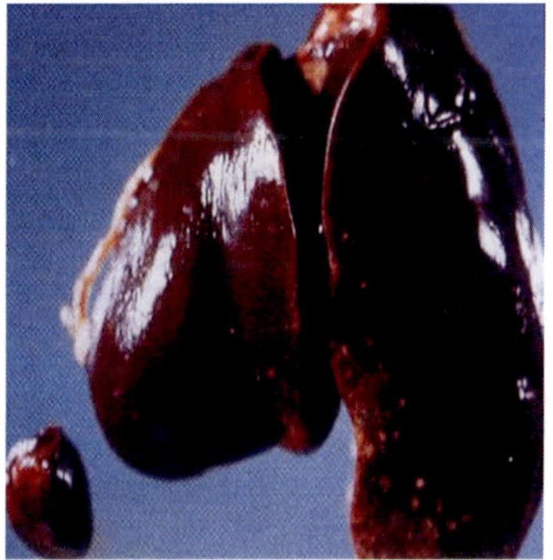

Fig. 59: DVE; multiple necrotic foci in the liver

49

Duck Virus Hepatitis (DVH)

DVH is a highly fatal infection of young ducklings. Lesions are primarily in the liver.

Etiology

Three different viruses are known to cause DVH.

- **DVH 1:** DVH 1 is an enterovirus in the family Picornaviridae. Serologic variants of DVH 1 have been reported. It first occurred in Long Island, N.Y. in 1949 and caused 95% mortality in 2-3 weeks old ducklings in commercial duck farms. DVH 1 is worldwide in distribution.
- **DVH 2:** DVH 2 is an astrovirus and has been exclusively reported in the UK since 1965. It affects ducklings up to 6 weeks.
- **DVH 3:** DVH 3 is a member of Picornaviruses but unrelated to DVH 1. DVH 3 has been exclusively reported in the USA. It affects ducklings up to 5 weeks.

The disease has no public health significance.

Epizootiology

Natural outbreaks have been reported in ducks only. DVH 1 is extremely contagious. The virus is excreted in the faeces of infected and recovered ducklings. Ingestion of contaminated material infects susceptible ducklings. The aerosol infection has also been observed. Egg transmission has not been proved. Wild birds have been incriminated as a mechanical carrier of the virus over short distances.

Clinical Signs

• DVH 1

The onset of the disease is very rapid, and all mortalities occur within 3-4 days. Affected ducklings stop movements and lie down with closed eyes. They may fall on sides with head backwards (Figure 60: opisthotonus position). Death comes within an hour after the onset of clinical signs. Mortality is inversely proportional to the age, the youngest ducklings less than a week old show the highest mortality (95-100%); ducklings 1-3 weeks have 50% mortality and mortality amongst ducklings over four weeks varies between 0 to 25%. No clinical signs are usually visible in older ducks.

• DVH 3

The clinical signs are similar to DVH 1, but the mortality is much low, never exceeding 30% in natural outbreaks.

• DVH 2

Clinical signs usually appear within four days after exposure and include convulsions and opisthotonus posture. All clinically positive ducklings die within 1-2 hours. Mortality in young ducklings ranges between 10 and 50%.

Lesions

All 3 viruses produce similar lesions. The liver is the primary organ involved. The liver is swollen and shows diffuse haemorrhages (Figure 61). Spleen is sometimes enlarged. Kidneys are swollen and congested.

- **Microscopically:** Typical coagulative necrosis appears in hepatic tissue. There is proliferation of bile ducts and chronic hepatitis in survivors.

Diagnosis

1) Sudden onset, short course, rapid spread and hemorrhagic hepatitis in young ducklings suggest DVH.
2) Virus isolation and identification of virus:

DVH 1 can be isolated in;

A. Chick embryo (8-10 days)

B. Duck embryo (10-14 days)

C. 1-day-old ducklings.

Serologic Tests

1) Virus neutralization test has been useful in virus identification, epidemiological surveys and vaccination response in DVH 1.
2) DVH 2 needs electron microscopy on liver or blood for diagnosis.

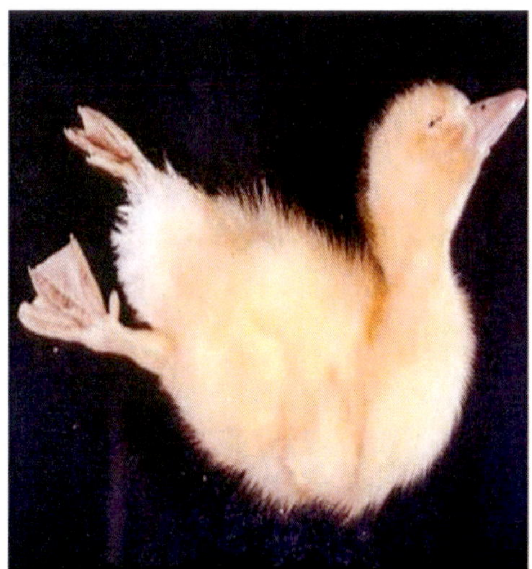

Fig. 60: Duck virus hepatitis (DVH); typical opisthotonos,

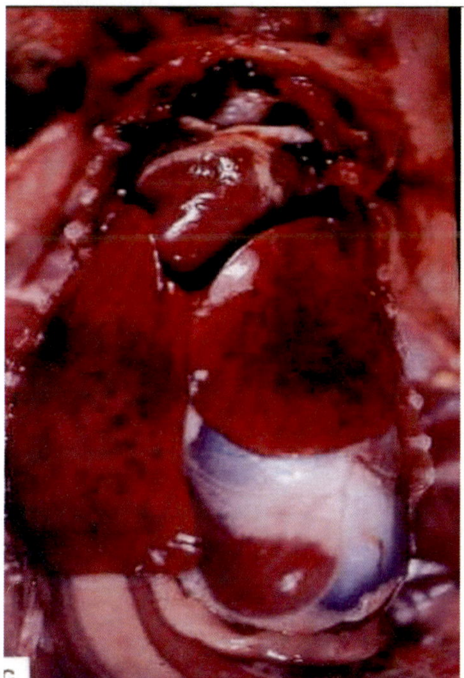

Fig. 61: DVH; massive hemorrhage and mottling of the liver

3) DVH 3 grows in duck embryos. It does not grow in chicken embryos and difficult to reproduce in ducklings.

Treatment

It is of no value.

Control and Prevention

• Immediate Action

Inoculate all susceptible ducklings I/M with duck viral antiserum. One inoculation is usually adequate.

• Long term action

Both live and inactivated vaccines are available. Ducklings are immunized using chicken embryo attenuated strain DVH type DVH1 Vaccine. Given in day-old ducklings by I/M or intranasal or foot web route, vaccine induces a considerable protection. Breeder ducks are vaccinated at 3-4 month intervals to maintain high antibody titer. Proper hygiene and sanitation methods are useful in controlling the outbreaks. DVH type 2 &3 Vaccines are still not available commercially.

50

Eastern Equine Encephalitis (Eee) Virus Infection

It is an acute disease of pheasants, chukars, partridges, turkeys, ducks, pigeons and wild birds. The viruses of EEE and WEE are of public health importance as they infect humans and occasionally cause fatal disease. The disease is further significant because of its link to disease in horses.

Etiology

The arboviruses are grouped into 12 different families. The five arboviruses causing disease in birds are Eastern equine encephalitis (EEE) virus, Western equine encephalitis (WEE) virus, Highland J (HJ) virus, Israel turkey meningoencephalitis (IT) virus and West Nile Virus WNV. The first three are in Togaviridae, and IT and West Nile Virus (WNV) are in Flaviviridae.

Occurrence

Most outbreaks of EEE in birds have been recorded in the USA especially in the states of Atlantic coast or in the upper Midwest. EEE affects pheasants primarily, however, outbreaks in pigeons, chukar partridges, finches, turkey and ducks have been reported. Outbreaks are mostly in mosquito season.

Transmission

Certain mosquitoes (Culiseta melnura) get infected with the virus from clinically positive birds or carrier birds. The virus may multiply inside the mosquitoes, but not an essential feature for transmission.

Infected mosquitoes transmit the infection through a bite to susceptible birds, horses or humans. Since birds have high virus titer during viremia as compared to other mammals, they are believed to play an important role in the epizootiology of the disease. Infection may also spread by cannibalism of viremic or dead birds.

Clinical Signs and Lesions

Many birds remain symptom-less carriers. Infected birds may show signs related to CNS derangement like ataxia, failing to stand up, paralysis, tremor and circling. Morbidity and mortality are high. In many birds (chicken, turkey, ducks, chukar & pheasants) lesions of nonsuppurative encephalitis, myocardial necrosis with mononuclear cell infiltration and or liver necrosis have been described. In rheas, EEEV produces haemorrhages and necrosis in the small intestine with widespread petechiae and necrosis in visceral organs. Also, EEEV produces necrotic lesions in ceca of rheas similar to intestinal spirochetes.

Diagnosis

Although clinical signs may be suggestive of the disease, isolation and identification of the virus do confirmation. Isolation can be done in chicken embryos, laboratory mice and tissue culture. Virus neutralization and complement fixation tests are useful in diagnosis.

Treatment

It is of no value.

Control and Prevention

Equine encephalitis vaccine may be used in birds. The dose is 1/10 the equine dose injected into the pectoral muscles, preferably at 5-6 weeks age.

The disease is a reportable disease in the USA.

• Western Equine Encephalitis

It is rarely associated with disease in birds; however, a few cases have been reported in Emu, pigeon and turkeys. It is mostly in the western parts of the USA and Canada. Clinical signs, diagnosis and control measures are same as for EEE.

• Highland J Virus Infection

HJ virus is antigenically related to WEE. It has been identified as the cause of disease in chukar partridge and turkeys. Clinical and pathologic characteristic of HJ virus resembles those of EEE virus. Israel Turkey Meningoencephalitis

Disease of turkey reported in Israel and South Africa.

• Affected turkeys exhibit neurological Signs

Progressive paresis and paralysis. Gross lesions include splenomegaly, myocarditis and catarrhal enteritis.

Control

1) Vaccination- with a live attenuated vaccine.
2) The reduction in insect vector population.

51

West Nile Virus (WNV)

WNV was first identified in the West Nile district of Uganda in 1937. Reported in Western Hemisphere for the first time in 1999, in New York City. The virus had until that time been found only in Africa, Eastern Europe, West Asia and the Middle East.

Etiology

WNV a flavivrus. It is closely related to St. Louise encephalitis virus found in the USA.

Transmission

No evidence of animal to animal, animal to person, or person to person transmission. Infection occurs through the bite of an infected mosquito. Mosquitoes become infected after taking a blood meal from a wild bird carrying the virus in the blood. Infected mosquitoes transmit infection to animals, birds and man. Mammals are generously "dead end" of the cycle.

Host and Disease

A. **Birds and other animals:** WNV has been isolated from over 63 species of birds, and many free ranging species (bat, raccoon). The virus is highly fatal in crows, blue jays and sometimes hawks. Most birds are most often found dead; therefore, description of clinical signs is not readily available nor have clinical signs associated with WNV infection in dogs, cats, bats, skunks, squirrels, rabbits and domestic birds been well described. It appears that although they may be infected, most members of these latter species may not develop clinical signs of disease.

A. Horses: are affected more often than other domestic animals. Many horses do not develop illness and many become ill and die with full blown encephalitis. The most common sign is weakness, usually in hind quarters. Weakness may be indicated by a widened stance, stumbling, leaning to one side and toe dragging. In extreme cases, paralysis may follow. Fever is sometimes noticed, accompanied with depression. Approximately 40% of cases of WNV encephalitis in horses proved fatal during the 1999 outbreak.

B. Humans: Disease is of zoonotic importance. Older people and immunocompromised persons develop severe illness with high fever, headache, coma, tremor, convulsion, paralysis and rarely death. In some cases skin rash and swollen lymph glands may be seen. Death rates associated with severe infection range from 3 to 15%, mostly among the elderly.

Diagnosis

1) Isolation of virus
2) Serology

Control

1) Controlling mosquitoes
2) **Vaccine:** The vaccine formed by removing key genes from dengue virus and replacing them with WNV genes, is under experiment in monkeys.
3) A vaccine is now available for horses. It is a reportable disease in the USA.

SECTION-4
Fungal Diseases

52

Aspergillosis (Brooder pneumonia)

Introduction

This is a disease mainly of the respiratory system affecting domestic poultry, wild birds and zoo birds. Systemic aspergillosis affecting visceral organs and other tissues of the bird's body is also reported. Reports are also available on eye and brain infections.

Epidemiology

1) *Aspergillus fumigatus* is the most pathogenic and frequently encountered species, of poultry and turkey. Cases have also been reported in waterfowl, psittacines, ratites, raptors, zoo birds etc. *Aspergillus glaucus* and *Aspergillus niger* may also be found in some cases, particularly in cutaneous lesions.

2) The disease is usually seen in young chicks in brooder house, where the mortality is very high, between 10 and 50%. Sporadic cases of the disease in adult birds are also seen. Faulty brooding and chilling predisposes to infection.

Clinical Signs

1) Many outbreaks are so acute that clinical signs are not observed and chickens die in high number.

2) Affected chicks show respiratory signs as gasping and accelerated breathing through the open beak (Figure 62). There is usually no respiratory sound as seen in other respiratory infections.

3) Chickens have increased thirst and fever. Some chicks appear sleepy.

4) In some outbreaks, diarrhoea and emaciation have been reported.

5) In turkey poults, in addition to the above clinical signs, nervous symptoms are also observed.

6) Serous excretions may also be seen from the eyes and nostrils.

Lesions

The lesions depend on the site of infection. It could be either localized or generalized throughout the body.

1) **Localized lesions** are usually observed in the respiratory tract affecting bronchi, trachea, air sacs and lungs. The lungs are most commonly involved. **In generalized infections** the lesions are seen in thoracic as well as abdominal cavity particularly involving the air sacs.
2) Lesions consist of nodules varying from pinhead to a millet seed size (Figure 63). The nodules have yellowish caseous center.
3) Grossly visible fungal mycelia may be present in the air passage and bronchi. In severely affected cases air passages are seen blocked with caseous pus. The fungi in the pus could be seen as dense green or black fur like structures.

Diagnosis

1) The history of respiratory problem in the brooder house along with typical accelerated breathing without any respiratory sound is indication of aspergillosis.
2) Postmortem lesions (typical nodules) are also suggestive of diagnosis. Care should be taken to differentiate caseous nodules seen in aspergillosis from that of pullorum disease in lungs of young chicks. This can be done by demonstration of fungus in fresh smears from cases of aspergillosis (Figure 64).
3) The culture of fungus can be done to confirm the diagnosis.

Treatment

1) Treatment with fungicides (nystatin, trichomycin, amphotericine B, Hamycin) has been reported in experimental flocks.
2) The treatment is usually useless. The whole flock be killed and disposed off properly.

Prevention and Control

Removing the cause does control of aspergillosis. Careful examination should be made for the source of infection and be removed immediately. Prevention depends on good hygiene, specially avoiding of damp feed and litter, cleanliness of drinkers and feeders, efficient ventilation of chicken houses and feed stores. Spraying of litter with antifungal drugs has been found beneficial. In outbreaks a 1:2,000 solution of copper sulfate is used as drinking water to prevent the spread of infection.

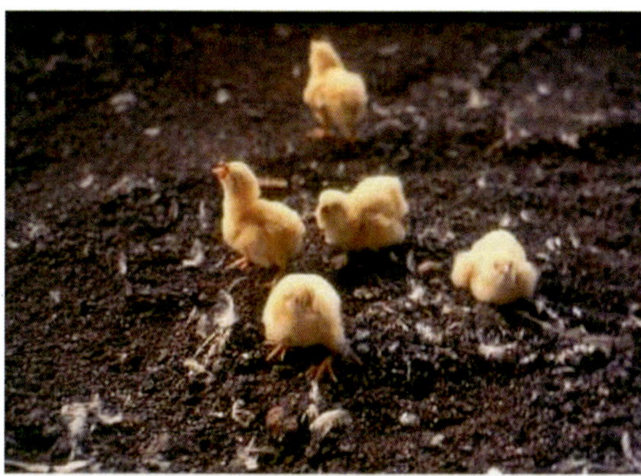

Fig. 62: Aspergillosis. Typical clinical signs (gasping)

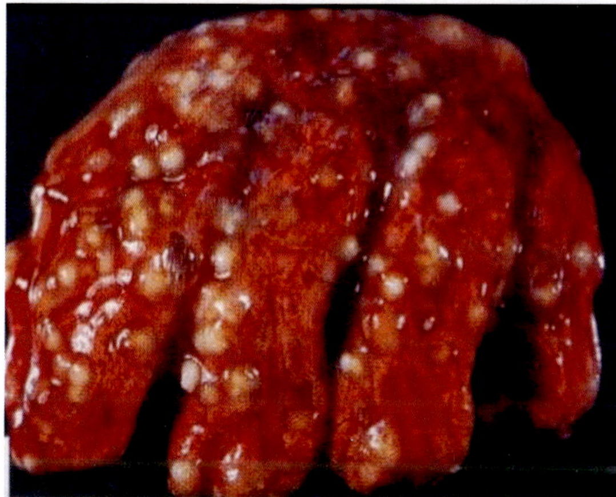

Fig. 63: Aspergillosis. White nodular lesions in the lung,

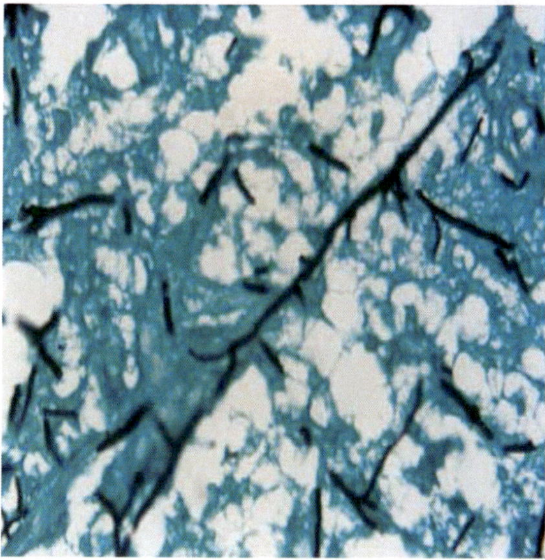

Fig. 64: Aspergillosis. Mycelia of fungus in the lesion

53

Candidiasis (Thrush; Mycosis of Digestive Tract)

Introduction

1) Serious outbreaks of thrush have been observed in chickens, pigeons, geese, turkeys, pheasants, quail, peacock and many other species of birds.

2) *Candida albicans* is the most commonly isolated fungus from the outbreak. Mucor spp. and Aspergilli were also found in some cases.

3) The outbreaks are associated with unhygienic conditions and nutritional deficiencies. Infection is more common in young birds up to 10 weeks of age. Morbidity is very high and mortality ranges from 10-75%. Clinical signs are not specific. Poor growth and ruffled feathers are only clinical signs.

Lesions

Lesions are mainly in crop but could be found in mouth, esophagus and occasionally in proventriculus. The mucosa of the affected digestive tract is thickened and has white circular raised ulcers, (Figure 65) giving an appearance of Turkish towel) which can easily be pealed off. Mucosa is covered with necrotic patches.

Diagnosis

Diagnosis can be made on clinical signs, gross lesions and isolation of yeast like fungus from the lesions.

Treatment

1) Treatment is of no use. Antifungal drugs can be tried with valuable individual birds. For the purpose:

   a. Mycostatin 200 g per ton of feed for 7-10 days and

b. Copper sulfate 1:2,000 in drinking water, given on alternate days for 5-7 days may be tried, to prevent the spread of infection during outbreak.

2) Preventive measures include correction of an unhygienic condition and over- crowding.

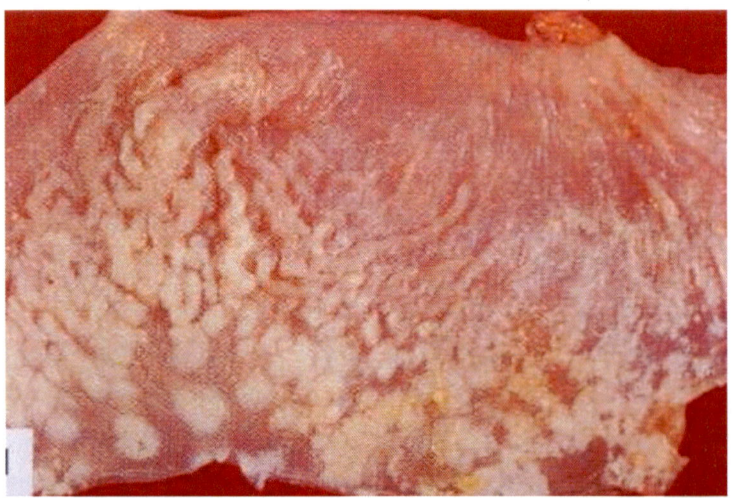

Fig. 65: Candidiasis. Lesions-typical ‘turkish towel” appearance

54

Cryptococcosis

Etiology

Cryptococcosis (KRIP-toe-cock-co-sis) is caused by the fungus, *Cryptococcus neoformans* (KRIP-toe-cock-kus knee-O-for-mans). It is found worldwide and primarily affects cats and people with weak immune systems.

Occurrence

Disease of can occur in humans and animals. The disease is not of significance in domestic poultry. However, a few cases have been reported from Pigeons, Canaries, Cockatoos, Macaws and African grey parrots.

Transmission

There have been no reports of direct animal-to-human transmission. People with weakened immune systems should limit their exposure to contaminated environments.

Clinical signs

The signs of illness will vary with the part of the body affected. Cryptococcosis can cause respiratory (lung) disease, skin lesions or infection of the nervous system (brain) or eyes.

Signs in these birds included weight loss, dyspnea and nasal exudate. Typical myxomatous lesions on the lung, liver and air sacs are observed.

Diagnosis

Isolation of *C. neoformans* from the droppings of Pigeons, Canaries, Fowls, Pheasants, Psittacines and other birds is of public health significance.

a) Culture of organism.

b) Histology of lesions : Mucicarmine stain is specific.

Prevention and Control

Precautions, such as wearing dust masks, should be taken when cleaning out old building/barns, since these areas may be contaminated with bird droppings. Always wash your hands properly after cleaning these areas.

55

Dermatophytosis (FAVUS)

It is a fungal infection of skin and the term favus is used for the disease in poultry. The disease is world wide in distribution.

Etiology

Microsporum gallinae, a fungus. The fungus is zoonotic. Lesions of ring worm are produced in humans in contact with infected birds.

Host Range

Observed in chicken, turkey, ducks, canaries and quails. Birds kept in small flocks usually in the backyard in free range, or semi intensive management and are predisposed to the infection.

Clinical Signs and Lesions

Usually, birds are seen healthy. Greyish white crusty lesions are observed mostly on un feathered comb, wattles and head. Lesions look as white flour has been sprinkled. When lesions extend to feathered part of the skin, there is a loss of hairs.

Diagnosis

1) Typical lesions are suggestive of diagnosis.
2) Fungus may be demonstrated in skin scrapings. Skin scraping can be mounted on the slide after treatment with 10% KOH and examined for fungal hyphae.
3) For confirmation, the fungus may be cultured.

Treatment and Control

Antifungal drugs ointment may be used externally for treatment of individual bird.

Segregate the affected birds to prevent infection to flock.

56

Mycotoxicosis

Diseases caused by toxic metabolites of fungi are called mycotoxicosis. It affects man and animals including birds. Fungi which grow on feeds and grains in an unfavorable environment mostly cause mycotoxicosis in birds.

AFLATOXICOSIS

Aflatoxicosis is caused by mycotoxin of aflatoxin group B1, B2, G1 and G2. *Aspergillus flavus* produces aflatoxin in feed and grains. The fungus can also grow in poultry litter and poultry house dust. Aflatoxin is produced in favourable temperature and humidity for the growth of fungi.

Clinical Signs and Lesions

1) In natural conditions it may take 2 weeks after the feeding of toxic feed, when the symptoms develop and mortality starts.
2) There are no specific clinical signs. However, affected flock may show loss of appetite, decreased feed intake and reduced growth. A few birds may show ataxia, lameness and spasm of neck muscles characterized by opisthotonus. Nervous signs are more common in ducks. In birds aflatoxins primarily cause damage to the liver and the clinical signs relate to liver damage. Affected birds develop impaired immune system. There is considerable mortality.
3) Lesions are mainly in the liver. The organ becomes tan to yellow with jaundice and haemorrhage. Kidneys are swollen. There may be haemorrhages in heart and other muscles. Microscopically liver shows fatty changes and necrosis.

Diagnosis

Gross and microscopic lesions in the liver are suggestive of aflatoxicosis but not pathognomonic. The feed may be analysed for the presence of toxins. Day-old ducklings may be fed on suspected feed sample; clinical signs in ducklings develop within a week.

OCHRATOXICOSIS

Toxic strains of *Penicillium viridicatum* produce ochratoxins. Disease produced by ochratoxin has been reported in pigs and chickens from Denmark, Sweden, Norway and Ireland.

Etiology

Toxigenic strains of *P. viridicatum* and other species of Penicillum and *Aspergillus ochraceus* produces ochratoxins.

Clinical Signs and Lesions

In birds, the clinical signs of reduced feed intake and mortality are observed. Lesions occur in liver and kidney. Kidneys are swollen. Microscopically nephrotoxic changes are present in kidneys. Visceral gout may also be present.

TRICHOTHECENE MYCOTOXICOSIS OCHRATOXICOSIS (Fusariotoxicosis)

Toxigenic species of *Fusarium* produces fusariotoxin on grains. More than 40 trichothecene mycotoxins have been identified, but most common are T-2 toxin and diacetoxyscirpenol.

Clinical Signs and Lesions

1) Disease has been reported in chickens, pigeons, ducks and geese.
2) Main clinical signs in birds are reduction in feed in take, depression and bloody diarrhea.
2) Lesions are extensive necrosis of oral mucosa and areas on the skin with gastrointestinal disease.

SECTION-5
Parasitic Diseases

57

Coccidiosis

The disease is worldwide in distribution and remains the major parasitic problem in the poultry industry. The problems occur principally in poultry maintained on deep litter.

Etiology

Coccidiosis of all classes of poultry is caused by one or more of the many species of coccidia of Eimeria species. In chickens nine main species are encountered. *Eimeria tenella, E. necatrix, E. maxima, E. acervulina, E. mitis, E. mivati, E. hagani, E. brunetti* and *E. preacox.*

Transmission

All coccidia involve digestive tract except for renal coccidiosis in geese and ducks. Infected birds shed coccidial oocysts in droppings. Oocysts sporulate on the soil to become infective. Ingestion of a large number of sporulated oocysts results in clinical disease.

In canaries - coccidium, *Isospora serini* multiplies by asexual cycle in the organs (liver, lung and spleen) and by sexual cycle in the intestinal mucosa. Liver and spleen are enlarged and mottled. The parasites are found in the cytoplasm of monocytes.

Coccidiosis in Chickens

• Mortality and Morbidity

1) Outbreaks rarely occur at less than 10 days of age. More common in chickens between 4 and 6 weeks old.

2) Mortality depends on species of coccidia, age of chickens and immunity of the host. Mortality varies from 1 to 40%.

Clinical Signs

1) Acute outbreaks: Birds do not drink or eat, show ruffled feathers, bloody droppings, high temperature and increased mortality.

2) Chronic coccidiosis: Show gradual weakness, loss of weight, decreased feed intake and decreased egg production. Mortality is negligible.

Lesions (depends on species of coccidia)

1) ***E. tenella*** **:** Cecal lesions; enlargement of ceca, thickening of its walls and blood in the lumen (Figure 66, 67).

2) ***E. acervulina*** **:** Mainly in duodenal loop, but occasionally extending to anterior 1/3 of the small intestine (Figure 68). Moderate pathogenic species. Lesions are white gray transverse ladders like areas in duodenum and upper jejunum (Figure 69).

3) ***E. necatrix*** **:** In the middle small intestine (Figure 70). Causes thickening of wall, severe cases show blood in the lumen. Lesions appear as small white yellow spots mixed with bright red petechiae, seen from serosal surface (Figure 71).

4) ***E. maxima*** **:** In the middle small intestine (Figure 72). Lesions comprise of thickening of the wall, ballooning of the intestine, intestinal lumen filled with blood or brownish blood mixed material (Figure 73).

5) ***E. mivati, E. hagani*** **and** ***E. praecox*** **:** Upper small intestine. Less pathogenic species, hence produce chronic lesions. Lesions comprise of thickening of the intestinal wall with severe catarrhal inflammation.

6) ***E. brunetti*:** Lower small intestine (Figure 74). Pathogenicity is rated after E. tenella and E. necatrix. Lesions are seen as extensive coagulative necrosis resulting in deep ulcers (Figure 75).

E mitis **:** Lower small intestine extending occasionally to ceca. It is less pathogenic species. Lesions consist of catarrhal inflammation.

Diagnosis

1) Clinical signs and gross lesions may be suggestive of coccidiosis.

2) Microscopic examination of fresh smears of intestinal material for developmental stages of coccidia may confirm the diagnosis.

3) The intestine is best examined by removing it completely from the bird and laying it out at its full length on a tray and proceeding as follows.

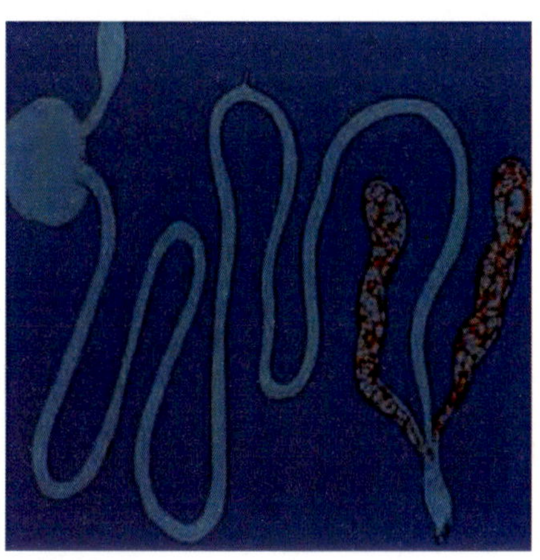

Fig. 66: Location of *E. tenella* infection; confined to ceca,

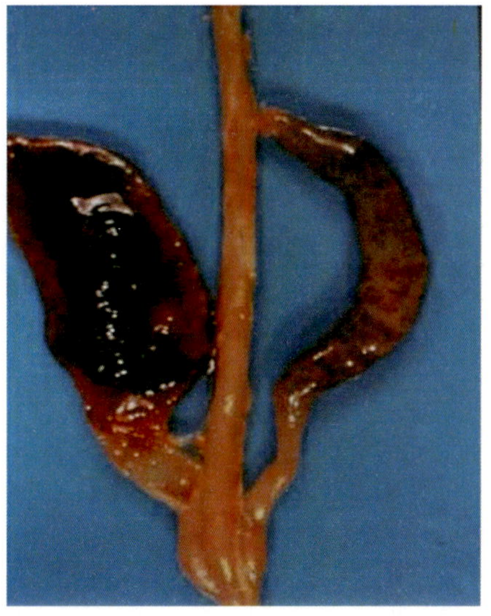

Fig. 67: *E. Tenella* infection; ceca distended with blood, petechial hemorrhages on serosa.

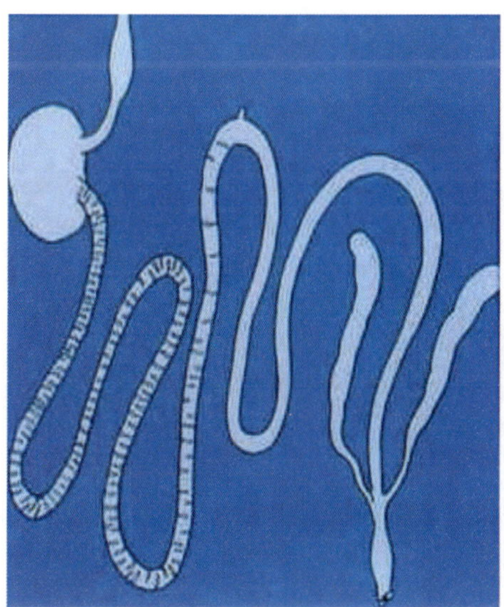

Fig. 68: Coccidiosis. Location of *E. acervulina* infections in the chicken- upper intestinal tract,

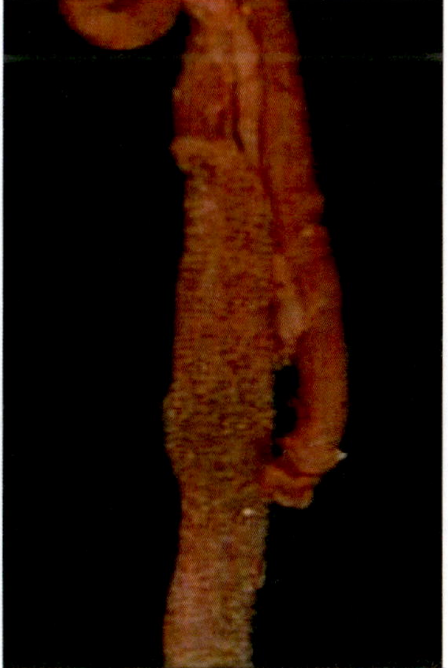

Fig. 69: *E. Acervulina* infection. Lesions are in the form of transverse bands, giving intestine a coated appearance

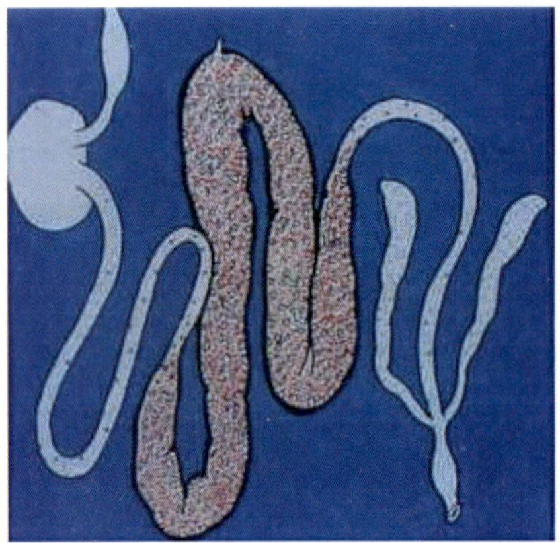

Fig. 70: Location of *E. necatrix* infection, usually mid intestine,

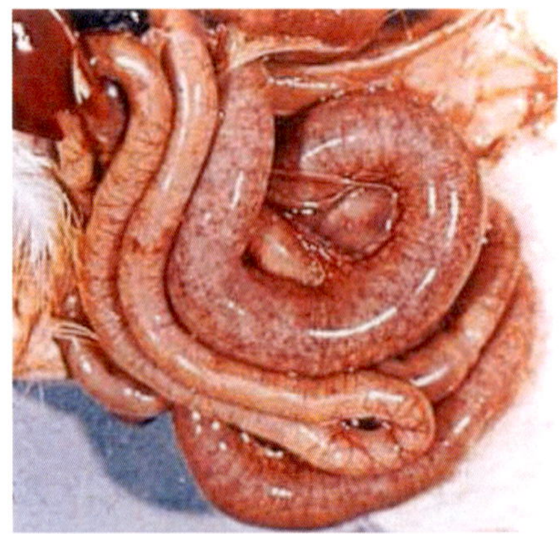

Fig. 71: *E. Necatrix* infection. Lesions consist of extremely ballooning and hemorrhage areas are clearly seen without opening the intestine; classic "salt and pepper" lesions on the serosal surface.

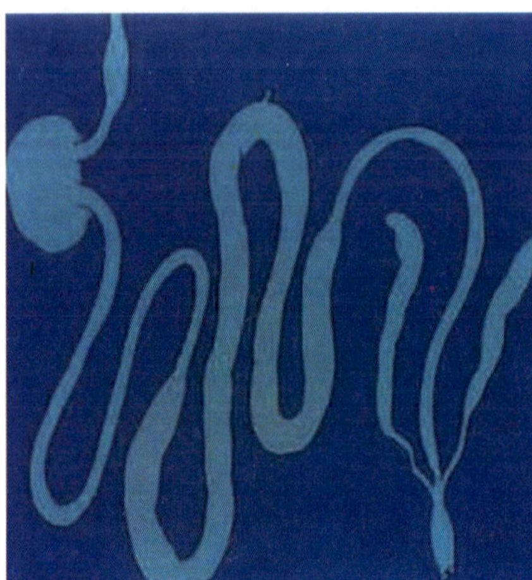

Fig. 72: Location of *E. maxima* infection, usually in the middle of the intestine but may extend to either side,

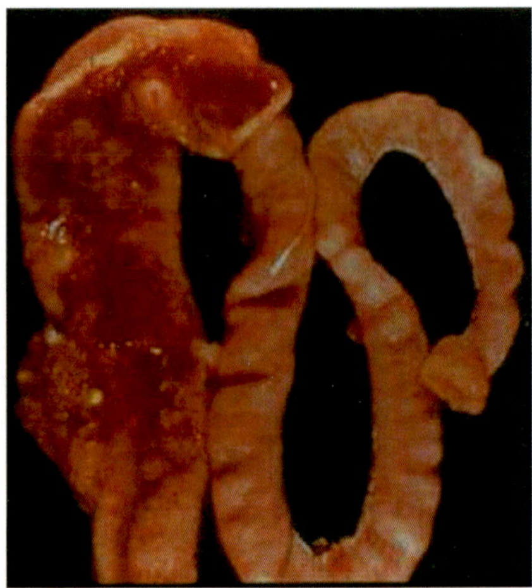

Fig. 73: *E. Maxima* infection. Lesions as red descrete hemorrhage on the serosal surface and orange mucus in the lumen.

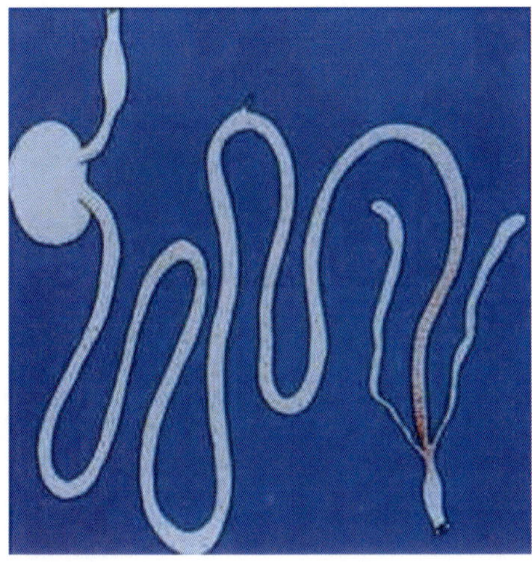

Fig. 74: Location of *E. brunetti* infection; lower small intestine

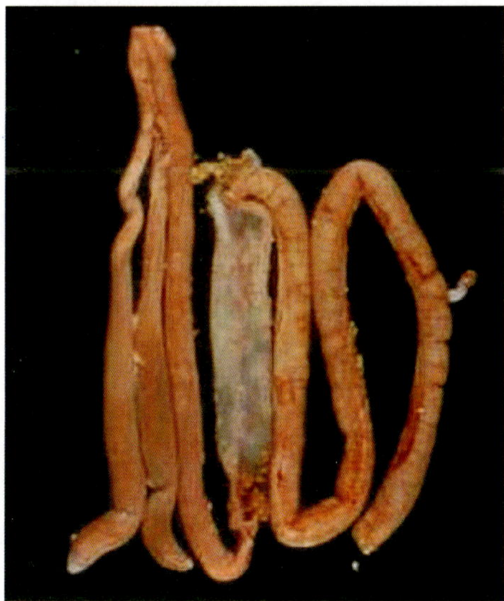

Fig. 75: *E. Brunetti* infection; lumen of lower small intestine contains hemorrhagic and mucoid content, ulcers seen in severe cases

a) Note the appearance of lesions on serous surface (outer surface): white spots or hemorrhages.

b) Open the intestine and note the type and the situation of the exudate and lesions (differential diagnosis chart).

c) Make smears of, 1. Exudate and 2. Epithelial layer (deep smears with scalpel blades).

Differential Characteristic of six species of Chicken Coccidia

	E.tenella	*E.necatrix*	*E.maxima*
Region of the intestine affected	Cecum	Middle small intestine	Middle small Intestine
Lesions	Blood white spots	Blood, thickened wall, White spots	Slight hemorrhage, pink exudate, Thickened wall
Virulence	+++	+++	+++

	E. brunetti	*E. mitis*	*E. acervulina*
Region of the intestine Affected	lower small intestine	lower small intestine	Upper small intestine
Lesions	Slight hemorrhage, Necrosis, ulcers	watery exudate	white transverse band watery exudate
Virulence	+++	++	+++

Treatment

Drugs for Treatment of Coccidiosis

Drug	Source	Treatment and duration	Withdrawl period (days)
Amprolium	Water	0.012-0.024% for 3-5 days	0
Pyrimethamine+ sulfaquinoxaline	Water	0.0015% pyrimidine compound+ 0.005% sulfaquinoxaline 2days on, 3days off, 2on	5
Sulfadimethoxine	Water	0.05% for 6 days	5
Sulfadimidine	Water	0.1% for 2 days, 0.055 for 4 days	10
Chlortetracycline	Feed	0.022% +0.8% calcium not more than 3 weeks	0
Oxytetracycline	Feed	0.22% + 0.5% calcium not more than 5 days	3

Water medication is usually preferred over feed medication for treatment.

• Anticoccidial drugs in broilers

Often a single drug will be used from day 1 to slaughter with a withdrawal period of 3 - 7 days. Shuttle or dual program is also sometimes used. Use of one product in Starter and other in Grower feed is called a shuttle or dual program. This program helps to reduce the build up of drug resistance.

• Programs used in breeders and layers

Pullets started on the floor and later reared, as cage layers do not need immunity to coccidiosis. They are given preventive medication as with broilers until they are moved to pens. Breeders and commercial layers kept on the floor should have immunity to coccidiosis. Immunity can be given by using a commercial product (coccivac) or by a light natural exposure. Vaccination or natural exposure is followed by use of a broad-spectrum anticoccidial drug in feed for 6-12 weeks.

Prevention and Control

1) Husbandry

a) Good management to prevent the warm moist condition in the poultry house which helps the development of coccidial oocysts.

b) Litter should always be dry near the drinkers.

c) Good ventilation will reduce the litter humidity and keep litter dry.

d) Clean litter should always be used for the fresh batch of chicks.

2) Use of Anticoccidial agents

Most farmers control coccidiosis by the preventive use of anticoccidials in the feed. Since coccidia soon become resistant to most anticoccidials, these are changed or used in combination. Exposure of chickens to a moderate number of coccidial oocysts (vaccine) combined with a use of anticoccidials protects the birds better if the anticoccidials are discontinued. However, some farmers prefer to keep chickens on anticoccidials to the entire period of chicken life.

3) Vaccination

A vaccine in the form of standard doses of sporulated oocysts of the various coccidial species is available. It is administered in the drinking water during the first 2 weeks of life. Since the "vaccine" serves only to introduce infection, the litter must be managed to allow oocyst sporulation. A wide range of anticoccidial is available on the market. Selection of the "best" is difficult. Some of the more popular ones include Amprolium (0.012%), monensin (0.01%), clopidol (0.02%) buquinolate (0.008%) and many others.

Coccidiosis in Turkeys

Pathogenic species: *E. adenoeides, E. meleagrimitis, E. dispersa*

Coccidiosis in turkeys effects poults mostly up to 2 months age. A bloody diarrhoea, a feature with many coccidial species in chickens, is not observed in turkeys. Flakes of blood may be present in faeces in turkeys with pathogenic coccidia.

- ***E. meleagrimitis*:** Affects 2/3 of the anterior intestine. Lesions include patchy areas of congestion and occasional petechial haemorrhage. It causes mortality and weight loss in young poults.
- ***E. dispersa*:** Affects middle 1/3 of the intestine but may extend to posterior part of the intestine. Lesions include the dilation of intestine with yellowish mucoid content. Occasionally it causes ulceration of mucosa and flakes of blood in the faeces. It is mildly pathogenic and causes diarrhea and weight loss.
- ***E. adenoides*:** Affects lower 1/3 of the intestine, mainly ceca. Lesions include edema and swelling of the intestinal wall. Clinical signs are liquid faeces with mucus and occasionally blood flakes.

Coccidiosis in Geese

- ***E. truncata*:** causes renal coccididiosis. Birds develop anorexia, weakness, diarrhoea with white faeces and nephritis with urate deposits.
- ***E. anseris*:** causes intestinal coccidiosis. Clinical signs include diarrhoea, weakness and mortality. Lesions are fibronecrotic enteritis in the middle and lower intestine.

Coccidiosis in ducks

- ***E. boschadis*:** mostly sporadic, a cause of renal coccidiosis. Species of Eimeria, Tyzzeria and Wonyonella may cause intestinal coccidiosis.

Coccidiosis in pet birds

A common protozoan disease in pet birds.

• Canaries

Isospora serini*; asexual cycle in spleen, liver and lung, and sexual cycle in the intestinal mucosa. Lesions consist of splenomegaly and hepatomegaly. Parasites are found in the cytoplasm of monocytes infiltrated in the lesion.*

• Psittacines

E. dunsingi and Isospora sp. – reported in lories, budgerigars, parrots, parakeets, causing enteritis.

• Passerines

E. lacarei cause enteritis in finches.

58

Cryptosporidiosis

Cryptosporidiosis is a protozoan disease.

Species

1) *C. meleagridis*: Infects small intestine.
2) *C. baileyi*: Infects digestive tract (bursa of Fabricius and cloaca), kidneys and respiratory tract.

Oocysts from infected birds are shed in faeces or respiratory secretions. Infection is through inhalation or ingestion of oocysts. Cryptosporidiosis has been reported in chicken, turkeys, quail, peafowl, pheasants, psittacines, waterfowl and finches. Avian species of Cryptosporidium have no public health significance.

Clinical Signs and Lesions

Parasites in the digestive tract cause diarrhea and fatal disease in young turkeys, quails and psittacines. In chickens, it causes weight loss. The intestine becomes dilated with foamy fluid contents. The respiratory infection causes swollen sinuses, coughing, sneezing, rales and nasal discharge. Lesions include greyish mucoid exudate on the mucosa of trachea, bronchi and nasal turbinates. Air sacs may be cloudy.

Diagnosis

Microscopic examination: Organisms can be demonstrated attached to the mucosa. They stain basophilic in H. & E. (2-5 um in diameter) and bright red with Carbol fuchsin. Faecal or respiratory specimens are submitted fresh in 10% formalin or 2.5% aqueous Pottasium. Dichromate solution.

Treatment

No effective drug is known for treatment or prevention.

Control

Stringent cleaning of premises with 10% formalin or 5% ammonia or undiluted commercial bleach is effective.

59

Histomoniasis (Black Head; Enterohepatitis)

Histomoniasis is a protozoan disease.

Etiology

Histomonas meleagridis.

Hosts

Mainly disease of turkey but has also been reported in chickens, peafowl, grouse, quail and gallinaceous birds.

Transmission

1) It is primarily by ingestion of ova of a cecal worm (Heterakis gallinae) containing the protozoan histomonas.
2) Ingestion of earth worms containing larvae of cecal worms in their tissues. Earth worm acts as transport host for cecal worm, and cecal worm serves as transport host for histomonas.
3) Ingestion of fresh faeces containing histomonas.

Clinical Signs and Lesions

In young turkeys, disease is fatal with 100% mortality. Symptoms appear in 2 weeks after the exposure. Initial signs include anorexia and yellow "sulfur coloured" faeces. Cyanosis of the head (black head) may be seen in a few turkeys. Older turkeys show gradual emaciation, depression, and drooping wings with head drawn close to the body. There is bilateral enlargement of ceca with the presence of caseous exudate in its lumen. Irregular round with depressed centre (saucer shape) necrotic areas of 1-2 cm size appears on the liver.

Diagnosis

Histomonad is flagellate in the cecal lumen but seen as amoeboid in tissues. Flagellates can be identified in cecal contents. Protozoa can be diagnosed by microscopic examination of the liver/ kidney tissue adjacent to the areas of necrosis.

Treatment

There is no approved medicine for food animals. Birds not for consumption are treated with metronidazole (30mg/kg body weight) given orally for 5-7 days.

Control

Good sanitation and strict biosecurity measures.

60

Trichomoniasis

Etiological Agent

Trichomonas gallinae, a flagellate protozoan. Strains vary in pathogenicity. The disease continues to be of significance in pigeons and doves. It has also been reported in raptors.

Transmission

In pigeons and doves transmission is through parent-nestling feeding. In raptors it is mainly through ingestion of infected prey. Chickens and turkeys may get the infection by consumption of contaminated water. Water gets contamination through secretion of infected or carrier birds.

Clinical Signs and Lesions

Infected squabs (baby pigeons) are depressed and die within 2 wk. of age. Mortality is high. Lesions are mostly in the mouth cavity but may extend to other visceral organs including liver and brain. Adult pigeons, doves and raptors have swollen, watery eyes. Because of lesions in the mouth they drool and make repeated attempts of swallowing. In cases of brain involvement, the signs of CNS disturbances are seen. Lesions in mouth cavity are typical caseous raised plaques.

Diagnosis

1) Typical clinical signs and lesions.
2) Demonstration of trichomonads in oral fluid, accompanied by the presence of typical caseous plaques in the mouth.

Differential Diagnosis

From lesions of pox and candidiasis.

Treatment

As for histomoniasis.

Control

1) Avoid mixing of pigeons, doves and susceptible birds.
2) Avoid feeding of infected birds to raptors.
3) Use strict biosecurity.

Giardia in pet birds

Giardia infects Budgerigars, Cockatiels, Macaws, Lovebirds, Cockatoos, Conures, Amazon Parrots. Syndrome in common in young birds which includes diarrhea, wasting and acute death. The zoonotic threat to humans is not proved.

Treatment

Metronidazole (25-35 mg/kg 1/m for 2 days); or 250 mg into 5002 drinking water.

61

Toxoplasmosis

Introduction

Chickens are considered one of the most important hosts in the epidemiology of Toxoplasma gondii infection because they are an efficient source of infection for cats that excrete the environmentally resistant oocysts and because humans may become infected with this parasite after eating undercooked infected chicken meat.

Poultry meat is an important part of cuisine, consumed widely all over the world; therefore, consumption of uncooked or not properly cooked poultry meat may pose a risk factor for *T. gondii* infection in humans or animals.

Etiology

Toxoplasmosis is caused by obligate intracellular protozoan *Toxoplasma gondii.* Cats are the definitive host for *T. gondii.* Mammals and birds serve as intermediate hosts. Toxoplasmosis is a zoonotic disease. Humans get infected by the handling of infected birds or by consumption of undercooked meat of infected birds. Chickens contribute to the *T. gondii* life cycle by acting as intermediate hosts or mechanical vectors.

Occurrence

Toxoplasma gondii has a worldwide distribution, and exposure to the organism is common. The main route of infection for chickens is assumed to be through ingestion of oocysts from soil.

Transmission

T. gondii infection can be transmitted if care is not taken to wash hands thoroughly after cutting meat and during cooking of meat; however, risk assessment studies have not been undertaken. Person-to-person transmission does not occur by direct contact, but transmission by organ transplantation or blood transfusion has been documented.

Clinical signs and lesions

Chickens are considered resistant to clinical toxoplasmosis. There are only a few reports of clinical toxoplasmosis in chickens worldwide. Microscopically, sciatic nerve neuritis, chorioretinitis and encephalitis were the main lesions.

The parasite affects mainly CNS but occasionally found in other visceral organs including, heart and skeletal muscles. It has been seen in canaries causing blindness. In chickens, although it is symptomless, sometimes may cause neurosis in the optic nerve leading to blindness.

Clinical signs in poultry include weight loss, inappetence, shrunken comb, drop in egg production, whitish diarrhoea, incoordination, trembling, opisthotonos (severe spasm in which the back arches), torticollis (twisting of the neck) and blindness. All chickens infected before eight weeks of age develop clinical signs. In older birds, infection can be asymptomatic (infected hosts show no symptoms) or latent (symptoms only develop under certain conditions).

Diagnosis

Animal meat and blood serum can be tested for *T. gondii* antibodies by modified agglutination test (MAT) and specific enzyme-linked immunosorbent assays (ELISAs).

Prevention and treatment

Good biosecurity and management procedures are the principle forms of control in commercial poultry flocks. Establish good rodent control and use separate staff for infected and uninfected flocks. Infected flocks should be depopulated as soon as possible after diagnosis is confirmed. Oocysts (the spore-like infective stage of the lifecycle that is passed in the faeces of the infected host) are resistant to detergents, acids and alkalis. Effective methods of disinfection include steam cleaning, ammonia, drying and heating (to 55°C for 24 hours). Concrete floors assist disinfection. Buildings should remain empty for four weeks after cleaning and disinfection.

Toxoplasmosis can be treated by using pyrimethamine at the rate of 0.5 mg/kg PO (oral) per day given in two equal doses every 12 hours for 7 – 10 days, with sulfadiazine at the rate of 30 mg/kg also given orally with the daily dose split in two equal doses every 12 hours, for the same time period.

62

Nematodes (Round Worms)

Introduction

A. Common species of nematodes encountered in poultry are:

a) ***Syngamous trachea*** **(in the respiratory tract)** large 2.00cm size live in the trachea and larger bronchi. Many species of domestic and wild birds are affected. Dyspnea, gasping and head shaking are main clinical signs. Treatment is difficult.

b) ***Ascaridia galli*** **(in the intestine)** They parasitize chicken, turkey, pigeon, quail and guineas. In younger birds parasites cause enteritis. In heavily infected birds clinical signs are emaciation and diarrhea.

1) ***Heterakis gallinarum*** **(in the intestine, mainly in cecum).** Affects mainly chicken, turkey, duck, goose, guinea fowl, pheasant and quail. Worms are small, white and thin up to 1.5 cm long. Worms are important because they are an intermediate host for *Histomonas meleagridis,* the cause of blackhead disease in turkeys. In heavy infested host it causes thickening and nodule formation in the cecal wall.

2) ***Capillaria species*** **(crop and intestine)** several species of genus *capillaria* infect crop, while others infect intestine. Worms are thin, thread like and vary from 6-25 mm. in length. They infect majority of domestic species of birds. Worms cause the thickening of mucosa of crop or intestine depending on the species involved. Clinical signs are diarrhea and emaciation and death.

3) **Tetrameres species (proventriculus)** They parasitize proventriculus of poultry. Adult worms are 3-18 mm. Clinical signs are diarrhea and anemia. They burrow the glands of the organ. Lesions are hemorrhages, and necrosis of the wall of the proventriculus.

B. Nematodes infections are mainly encountered in backyard flocks but are less frequently found under intensive conditions. However, severe parasitism may occur in floor reared layers/breeders.

C. They cause nonspecific sings such as general unthriftiness, retarded growth and lowered production. Affected birds show loss of bloom and have ruffled feathers. A few heavily affected birds may die.

Control

1) Control is by treatment with anthelminthics in either feed or water. In layers housed on deep litter and in backyard flocks one-day treatment every two months may be necessary.

2) Treatment with anthelminthics should be followed by a course of antibiotics and vitamins.

3) Piperazine salts are used for treatment. Single dose of 50-100mg/bird or 0.2- 0.4% in feed or 0.1-0.2% in drinking water is enough. Other drugs like Phenothiazine, Hygromycine B and Coumaphos are also in use for the treatment of round worms. Phenothiazine controls cecal worms at 0.5g/bird, one-day treatment. Hygromycin B 0.001% in feed, controls ascarids, cecal worms and *Capillaria* sp. Coumaphos used in feed at 0.003% for 10 - 14 days mainly for *Capillaria* sp.

63

Tapeworms (Cestodes)

Introduction

1) Various genera of tapeworms are found in poultry. They are:
   a) *Raillietina* spp.
   b) *Choanotaenia* spp.
   c) *Davainea* spp.
   d) *Amebotaenia* spp. and
   e) *Hymenolepis* spp.
2) Tapeworms mainly parasitise the small intestine. Tape worms deprive the bird of its nutrition and cause weight loss and decreased egg production.
3) Out of 3 species of *Raillitina, Raillietina echinobothrida* is one of the pathogenic species as it produces granuloma at its attachment site (nodular disease).
4) They all require intermediate host for their development.
5) Intermediate hosts are common houseflies, ants, beetles and grasshoppers, which makes control of tapeworms difficult.

Diagnosis

Tape worms and their identification can be done on the following cirtarioa.

1) Size and shape of scolex
2) Size and shape of eggs
3) Study of individual proglottids
4) Features of whole parasite.

Control

1) The use of insecticides to control intermediate hosts in poultry houses is suggested.

2) Treatment with specific tapeworm anthelmenthics is reported as successful. Butynorate (0.07 to 0.14%) in feed is effective against tapeworms.

64

Blood Borne Parasite

HAEMOPROTEUS

Host

Infection with *Haemoproteus* species is host specific.

H. meleagridis – domestic poultry and pet birds

H. olumbae in pigeons

H. nettionis in waterfowl.

Transmission

Biting flies and midges act as vectors.

Clinical Signs

In majority of the infected birds clinical signs, are inapparent. In small proportion of birds emaciation, depression, anemia and anorexia are observed. Observation of gametocytes with pigment granules in blood smears stained with Giemsa or Wright's stain is diagnostic.

LEUKOCYTOZOA

Birds are main host of leukocytozoan. Many species of the parasite have been identified and they are host specific. The disease is seen in acute and chronic form. Acute disease mostly occurs in young birds and chronic form in older birds. Black flies and Culicoid midges act as vector, where parasite undergo sporogony.

Clinical Signs and Lesions

1) Sudden onset of depression, weakness and anemia are seen in many infected birds.
2) The birds in acute stage die or may recover.
3) In chronic phase birds show hepatomegaly and splenomegaly.

Diagnosis

Presence of gametes in erythrocytes or leukocytes in blood smears stained with Giemsa or Wright's stain is diagnostic.

65

Ectoparasites

LICE

Introduction

Lice are common ectoparasites of birds. There are many species of bird lice and are found on chicken, turkey, guinea fowl, duck, goose and pigeon. Lice species prefer a different part of the body. Most of them are straw colour and measure 1-10 mm. Lice from one host can parasitise another host if they are in close contact. For example, a louse from chicken can parasitise guinea fowls kept on the same premises. Hence, the species of lice is determined if cross contamination from another species is suspected. Lice are not highly pathogenic to mature birds. However, severe lousiness may lead to weight loss, as well as low production and death.

Control

1) Lice tend to increase during autumn and winter, so flocks are examined for lice on a regular basis preferably two times a month. Treatment can be by dusting or spraying of the insecticide. Dusting may work well in small-scale units. Dusting is applied to litter, giving particular attention to cover under roosts, feeders and nest boxes. Dusting of individual birds may also be carried out.

2) In large units and caged layers, spraying is a method of choice. High-pressure sprays (125pounds/inch2) are most suitable.

3) Insecticides are available as dust, wettable powder, emulsifiable concentrates and water dispersible liquids. The last three are intended for spray. Care should be taken that feed and water are not contaminated.

4) Common insecticides in use are malathion, Coumaphos, Carbaryl and many others. Label directions should be strictly adhered to for the type of the insecticide you choose.

5) The treatment should be twice on a 7-10 days interval, to control the lice that hatch after the first treatment.

BUGS

Introduction

Bugs are common blood sucking parasites of birds. The most wide spread of these is a common bedbug. It is most prevalent in subtropical climates and attacks most mammals including humans and poultry. The other important bird bug is poultry bug. Feeding usually occurs at night. The bugs become engorged within 10 minutes, then hide in cracks and crevices of the poultry houses. Heavy infestation may cause birds anaemic. Swelling and itching usually follow bites.

Control

1) Control is accomplished by thorough cleaning of the houses, reducing hiding places for the bugs and spraying with insecticides as for lice.
2) Fumigation is helpful to flush the bugs from their hiding places.

FLEAS

Introduction

1) Fleas are parasites in the adult stage. Adult fleas are reddish brown about 1.5 mm long. Many species of fleas have been found on birds. They infect mammals as well.
2) Heavy infestation causes irritation and blood loss, especially in young birds, which may die.
3) Production is lowered in older birds.

Control

Control measures include removal of infected litter and spraying of the house with insecticides to kill immature fleas.

MITES

Introduction

1) Mites are most economically important external parasite of poultry.
2) The family Dermanysidae include the chicken mite, northern fowl mite and tropical fowl mite.
3) They are bloodsuckers and can run rapidly on skin and feathers.

a) Chicken mite *Dermanyssus gallinae* (red mite, roost mite, poultry mite)

Chickens are the commonest host but may occur on turkeys, pigeons, canaries and many species of wild birds. Humans may also be attacked. Mites are tiny 0.7 x .04 mm in size. They not only produce anaemia but lower production but are also known to transmit spirochetes and other disease agents. These mites often can be found under loose clods of manure, under slats in brooding house, in nests or in cracks and crevices. They are seen as tiny red to blackish dots often clustered together. They can be found on the shanks of birds.

b) Northern fowl mite *(Ornithonyssus sylvarum)*

Commonest parasite of poultry. Unlike chicken mite, it can be easily found on birds in the day as well as the night. In heavy infestation, feathers are blackened, and skin is scabbed and cracked around the vent. Heavy infestation reduces reproductive potential in males, egg production in females and weight gain in young birds.

c) Tropical fowl mite

Hosts include poultry, pigeons, sparrows, myna birds and humans. This parasite can pass entire life cycle on the host. It is less pathogenic.

d) Depluming mite

1) These burrow into the epidermis at the base of feather shaft and cause intense irritation and feather pulling in chickens, pigeons, geese and pheasants. Affected birds lose weight and show lower production.

2) Control is by prompt isolation of affected birds and disinfection of houses. The affected birds should be treated by dipping individual birds in a mixture of sulfur 60g with soap 30g in 4 litres of warm water.

e) Feather mites

1) Feather mites are rarely found on modern chicken farms. Economic damage by these mites is rare. However, feather loss and crust like dermatitis in mite infested body region (lower legs, skin of the comb and wattles) are reported.

2) No specific control measures have been described. Disposal of affected birds and disinfection of poultry houses are advised.

f) Scaly leg mite

1) It is rare in modern poultry, but when occurs it is in older birds. Mites usually tunnel into the tissue under the scales of the legs. The exudation in affected part causes thickening and encrustation.

2) For control general cleaning and disinfection of poultry houses is advisable. Individual birds may be dipped twice (10-day interval) in kerosene, crude oil, mineral oil or coated with vaseline. After loosening of the scale, the legs should be dipped in warm acaricide solution.

3) Ivermectin (200 mg/kg body weight) given subcutaneously or cutaneously, is the drug of choice. Three treatments with an interval of 2 weeks is a usual protocol. Complete disinfection of cages is needed for prevention of re-infection.

Control

1) Chicken mite, Northern fowl mite and tropical fowl mite may be controlled by the same insecticides applied to birds, litter, nests and walls of the facility.

2) Birds can be treated with any insecticides but ensure that the skin is wet.

   Of lesser importance are members of other mite families that bore into the skin or infect various internal organs/passages.

TICKS

Introduction

Fowl ticks ***(Argas persicus)***

1) Soft-bodied ticks are the most important ticks of poultry. The genus consists of three species. All stages may be found hiding in cracks and crevices during the day. Larvae can be found on the birds because they remain attached and feed for 2-7 days. Nymphs and adults feed at night. Red spots can be seen on the skin where the ticks have fed.

2) Fowl ticks produce anemia, weight loss, depression, toxemia and paralysis. Egg Production decreases. Fowl ticks, also are capable of transmitting many important poultry diseases like spirochetosis, aegyptinellosis and fowl cholera.

Control

Control is accomplished by cleaning the walls, ceiling, cracks and crevices with insecticides preferably using high-pressure sprayers.

SECTION-6
Deficiency Diseases

66

Vitamin Deficiency

Vitamin A

Source of Vitamin

Berseem, legumes, alfalfa or other grass meal, fish oils, yellow corn, palm oil, commercial Vitamin A concentrate

Recommended per Kg of feed

a) Chicks, growing pullets 1500 I.U.

b) Laying and breeding hens 4000 I.U.

c) Turkeys (All age groups) 4000 I.U.

Clinical symptoms and pathological picture of deficiency

Vitamin A is essential for healthy development and repair of all epithelial structure and the bones. Lack of vitamin in young chicks results in reduced growth, ruffled feathers; lack of yellow pigmentation in shanks and beaks; keratinization of skin; lachrymation, swelling around the eyes and deposition of cheesy material under the eye lids; pustules in the mouth, oesophagus (Figure 76), crop and respiratory tract. Deficiency in mature chickens develops more slowly and results in the drop in egg production, decrease in the hatchability and high mortality of chicks during the first two weeks.

Vitamin D

Source of Vitamin

Fish oils, vitamin D3, sunlight, and irradiated animal sterols.

Recommended per Kg of feed

a) Chicks & growers: 200-500 ICU

b) Laying and breeding hens: 500 ICU

c) Turkeys (All age groups): 900 ICU

(ICU: International chick unit)

Clinical symptoms and pathological picture of deficiency

Vitamin D is required for normal absorption and metabolism of calcium and phosphorus. Deficiency produces rickets and osteoporosis.

Signs of rickets in growing chickens are the disinclination to walk, leg weakness with a lame stiff legged gait, retardation of growth; enlargement of hock joints. Other signs include swelling and beading at the end of ribs (Figure 77) marked softening of skeleton including beak (Figure 78) bending of sternum and spinal column and thickening of extremities of long bones.

In laying chickens prompt reduction of both egg production and hatchability, thin or soft shelled eggs, and rubbery breast bones.

Vitamin E

Source of Vitamin

Cottonseed oil, peanut oil, wheat germ oil, soybean oil and grains. Only stabilized fat should be used in the feed. Bad storage of feed destroys Vitamin E.

Recommended per Kg of feed

a) Chicks, growers and hens 10-15 I.U.

b) Turkeys (All age groups) 10 I.U.

The requirement of Vitamin E will vary depending upon the type and level of fat in the diet and level of selenium.

Clinical symptoms and pathological picture of deficiency

The deficiency of vitamin E produces encephalomalacia, exudative diathesis and muscular dystrophy in chicks. It is also required for normal reproduction and embryonic development.

Encephalomalacia is a nervous derangement. It is usually seen between 2nd and 5th week of the chicks life characterized by ataxia, sudden prostration with legs outstretched and toes flexed, lack of coordination in movement, walks in a drunken fashion, lateral twisting of the head with paralysis, and falling on its back (Figure 79), death soon follows. Lesions are confined on cerebellum; seen as swollen cerebellum, haemorrhages and areas of necrosis (Figure 80).

Exudative diathesis is an oedema of the subcutaneous tissue in the abdominal region. The oedema fluid is greenish blue in colour. The chicks stand with their legs apart. Seen in chicks between 5 and 11 weeks of age.

Muscular dystrophy, seen between 4 and 8 weeks of age, is degeneration and necrosis of muscle fibers, seen as white streaks in normal pink colored muscles (Figure 81). The condition affects all muscles of body including muscles of heart and gizzard.

In mature chickens no outward signs of deficiency of Vitamin E appear even after a prolonged period. However, deficiency leads to loss of fertility in males and poor hatchability in breeding hens.

The role of this vitamin is interrelated with selenium for prevention of exudative diathesis. In another role it is interrelated with selenium and cystine for prevention of muscular dystrophy (see selenium).

Chickens respond in a matter of a few hours to oral administration of this vitamin.

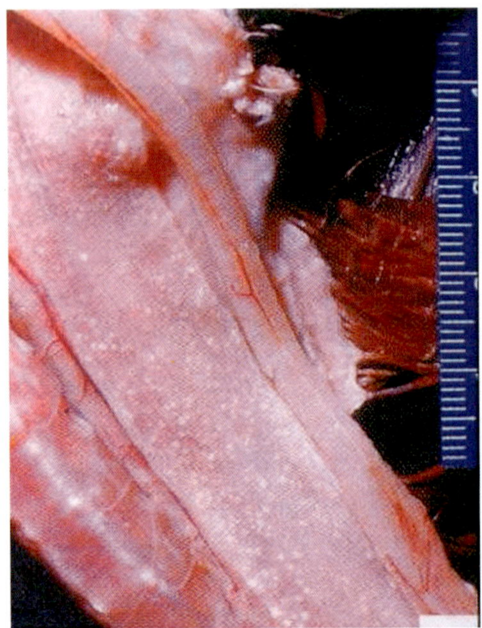

Fig. 76: Vitamin A deficiency; distended impacted mucosal glands resembling pustules in the esophagus.

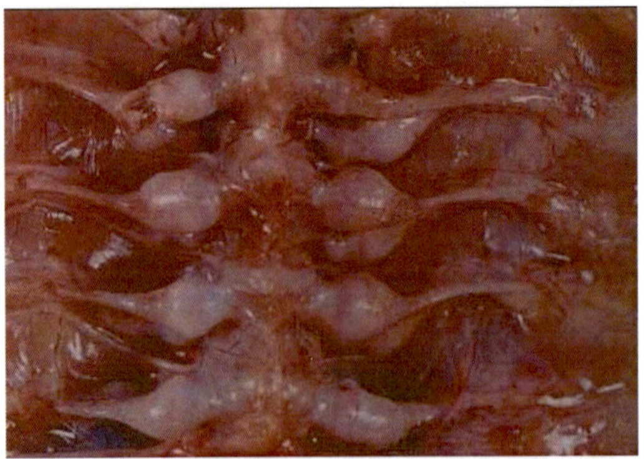

Fig. 77: Vitamin D deficiency; lesions of rickets rosary (beading of rib head),

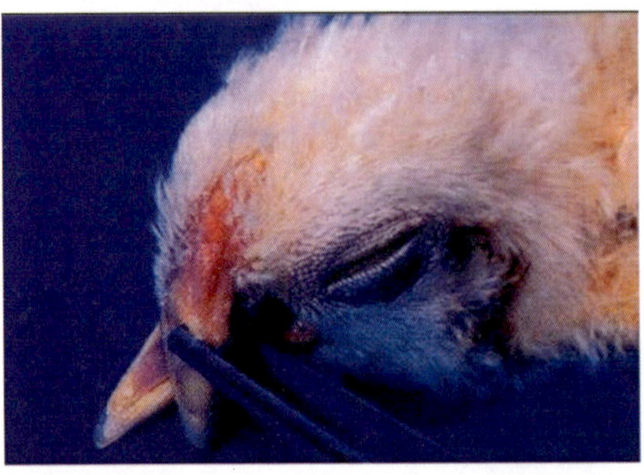

Fig. 78: Vitamin D deficiency; softening and bending of the beak

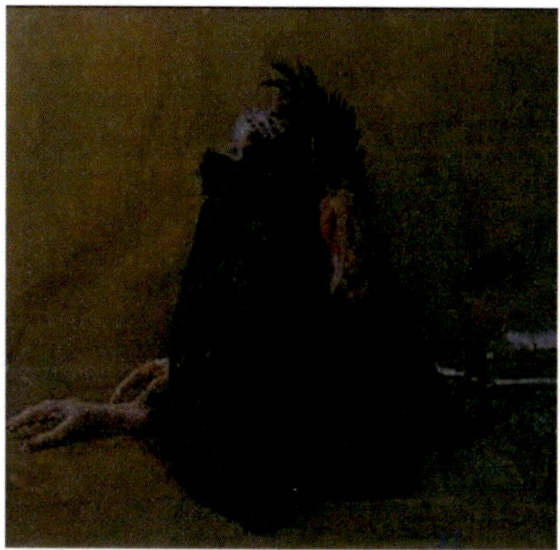

Fig. 79: Vitamin E deficiency; opisthotonos in a 5 weeks chick.

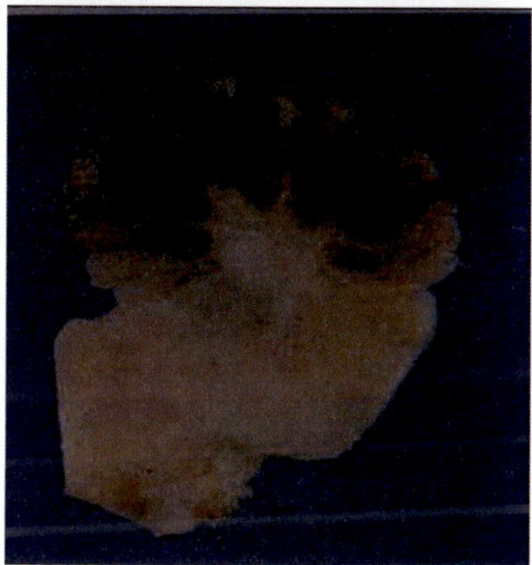

Fig. 80: Vitamin E deficiency; encephalomalacia- extensive hemorrhage of the cerebellum.

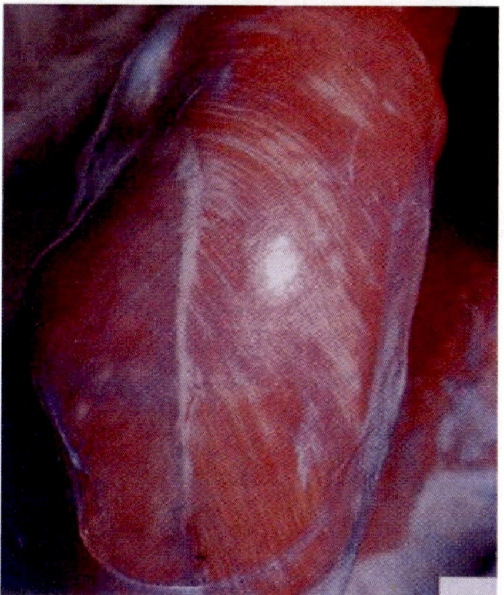

Fig. 81: Vitamin E deficiency; nutritional myopathy showing streaks of degenerated muscles

67

Mineral Deficiency

CALCIUM & PHOSPHORUS

Source of mineral

Soluble grits (Limestone grits containing chiefly CaCo3) which is soluble in acid medium of crop. It differs from insoluble grits (gravel, granites, sand etc.) which acts only mechanically in the gizzard.

Recommended per Kg of feed

a) For growing chicks: Ca 1%; Ca/P ratio 2:1

b) For poults: Ca 2%; P 1%; Ca/P ratio 2:1

c) For laying hens and Turkeys: Ca 2.25%; P 0.75%; Ca/P ratio 3:1

Clinical symptoms and pathological picture of deficiency

In growing birds the signs are very similar to those of Vitamin D deficiency. Birds become lame with a stiff-legged gait and show retardation of growth and ruffled feathers. The bones are rubbery and the joints tend to be enlarged. Rickets develop and some of the birds may show paralysis.

In laying birds the skeleton is gradually depleted of these minerals becoming osteoporotic. In marked deficiency this may lead to paralysis. The bones are thin, deformed and more prone to fractures. A few thin-shelled eggs with lowered production and hatchability are produced.

MANGANESE

Source of the mineral

Wheat bran and wheat products, alfalfa meal, soybean meal and manganese compounds.

Recommended per Kg of feed

a) Chicks and poults: 55 mg.

b) Hens and Turkeys: 30-35 mg.

Clinical symptoms and pathological picture of deficiency

The deficiency in young chickens causes perosis, which is malformation of the hock joint. The main features, similar to choline deficiency, are swelling and flattening of the hock joints, twisting and bending of the distal end of the tibia and of the proximal end of the metatarsus and finally slipping of the gastrocnemius tendon from its condyles (Figure 82). A shortening of the legs, wings and spinal column is apparent.

In adult chickens a diet deficient in manganese tends to show reduced egg production, hatchability and viability of chicks. The shells of their eggs become thinner and less resistant to breakage due to poor calcification of the shell. Embryonic mortality usually starts after the 10th day of incubation and dead embryos show bone abnormalities characterized by short thickened legs, short wings, parrot beak, a globular contour of head, protruding abdomen.

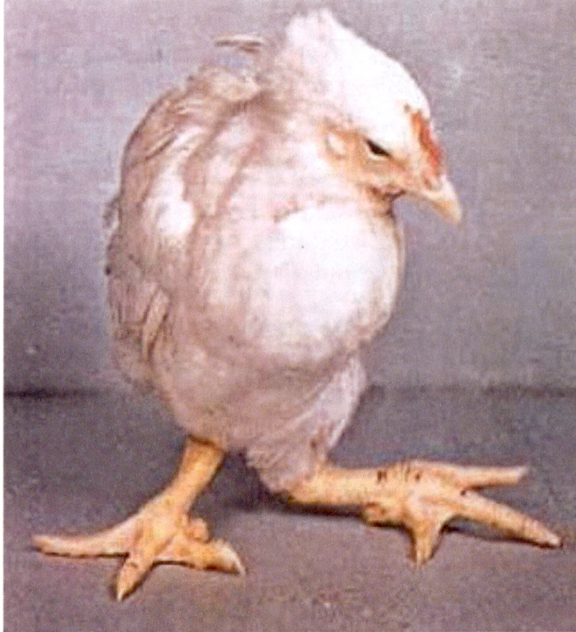

Fig. 82: Manganese deficiency; perosis: The common sign is deformity of the leg bones

SELENIUM

Source of the mineral

Feed grown on high selenium soils are good sources of selenium.

Dried brewer's yeast and a chemical compound (sodium selenite) are also good sources (see also Vitamin E).

Recommended per Kg of feed

Chicks and poults: 0.15 to 0.2 mg.

Caution

As little as 10 mg of selenium per kg of feed is toxic.

Clinical symptoms and pathological picture of deficiency

Deficiency in growing chickens causes exudative diathesis, usually between 5 and 11 weeks of age. The subcutaneous edema results in weeping of the skin seen on the inner surface of thighs and wings. Hemorrhages on the musculature, intestine and other visceral organs may also be noticed. Edematous fluid in the subcutaneous part and abdomen may be blood tinged.

In laying hens deficiency affects egg production.

SECTION-7
Miscellaneous Disorders

68

Bumble Foot (Pododermatitis/ Planter absces)

Pododermatitis or bumble foot has many causes including excess weight bearing from obesity or unequal weight bearing between the two feet as a result of lameness of one foot, causing less weight to be placed on that foot and more on the contralateral foot, or from abnormal abrasions of the plantar surface from inappropriate substrate (too sharp or rough, wire, etc.), decreased blood supply to the foot (sometimes from lack of exercise), trauma, or standing for prolonged periods of time, especially in ducks that are not provided with adequate swimming opportunities.

Bumble foot is commonly seen in waterfowl under one or more of the following conditions; obesity, hard substrate, lack of access to water to swim in, malnutrition and underlying disease.

This is localized infection of the feet. It is seen as bulbous swelling of the footpad and surrounding tissues. It appears usually after an injury to the foot pad and causes lameness in one or both feet. Pododermatitis is divided into varying grades depending on the literature source used, but generally includes mild, moderate, and severe grades with the severe grades including osteomyelitis. Infection by various bacteria commonly occurs and superficial wounds may not be present. Sometimes ulcers are formed on the planter surface of the foot. The layers become lame and production lowers, sometimes completely stops. On opening the swelling a foul smelling thick pus is found. The condition is more common in heavy breeds. Early surgery and antibiotic therapy may control the condition. Removal of high roosts reduces the incidence.

Carcasses with lesions from which staphylococci or other bacteria are isolated also have liver discoloration, but frequently turkeys with liver discoloration do not have demonstrable osteomyelitis or associated lesions, or bacteria cannot be isolated from the lesions.

Bumble foot can be treated by antibiotics and anti-inflammatory drugs and birds should not keep in the iron cages.

69

Cage Layer Fatigue (Osteoporosis)

Cage layer fatigue is a term used to describe leg weakness and acute deaths in chickens in cages, and is caused by inadequate calcium, phosphorus and Vitamin D levels in the blood stream. Calcium is required for muscle function, bone formation, and egg shell formation. This condition may be seen even in floor birds under certain conditions. It is seen most often in young hens early in production.

1) As the name implies, the major feature of the condition is reduced bone structure in laying chickens kept in cages.
2) Initial clinical signs consist of paralysis, later becoming depressed and dying of dehydration. On postmortem examination, bones are easily broken; fractures may be found in leg and wing bones. Ribs may be bent at the junction of the sternum and vertebral components. The sternum is often deformed. Parathyroid glands are enlarged.
3) Although diet poor in calcium, phosphorus and Vitamin D have been shown to produce similar skeletal changes, the condition restricted to birds kept in cages suggests to the lack of exercise causing poor skeletal development.

Affected birds removed from the cages and fed on balanced ration recover in a week.

70

Stunting Runting Syndrome

Introduction

Although the causative agent for the condition has not been identified, experimental studies indicate the association of parvovirus and or Astrovirus. Under experimental conditions, the virus induces clinical signs only in fast growing broiler chickens. The clinical signs, based on experimental inoculation of chickens, consist of watery or mucoid mustard yellow colour diarrhoea within 3-5 days after infection. Chickens become stunted, and a variable number of such chickens die during 10 and 20 days. Pronounced weight loss is in around four week's age. The mortality is low (5 - 10%) however, the morbidity is very high (50 - 80%).

Gross Lesions

Gross lesions consist of reduced body size with the white, pale colouration of small intestines. The pancreas is white, firm and shrunken.

Diagnosis

1) Uneven growth of broiler chickens can be an indication of parvovirus infection.

2) Diagnosis can be confirmed by demonstration of virus particles by an electron microscope, or by indirect immunofluorescence assay performed on smears of the duodenum.

Prevention and Control

Since no particular method is available for the control, general hygiene measures should be followed.

71

Ascites Syndrome (Water belly, Right ventricular failure, Hypertension syndrome)

Introduction

1) The condition has been reported the world wide in growing broiler chickens.

2) The affected birds show clinical signs usually during 4 - 5 weeks of age. The clinically affected birds are smaller, listless with ruffled feathers, pale head and shrunken comb. Severely affected birds have distended abdomen, which restricts their normal movement. Death may occur suddenly, and not all the broilers which die of the condition have ascites. The incidence of the disease varies between 2 to 20%.

3) Gross lesions include ascites, right side cardiac enlargement and liver damage. There is a variable amount of clear yellow fluid and clot of fibrin in the abdomen. In the majority of cases, fluid volume exceeds 300 ml. The liver varies from congested or mottled to shrunken with a greyish capsule and irregular surface. There is mild to marked hydropericardium. There is marked right ventricular dilation. The lungs are extremely congested and edematous.

4) The condition is caused by increased pressure in the pulmonary arteries when heart tries to pump more blood through the lungs to meet the body's oxygen requirement, in fast growing broilers.

5) Factors, which increase oxygen demand, are:

    a) Cold

    b) Bad ventilation

    c) Interference with blood flow through the lung

d) Reduced oxygen carrying capacity of the blood (carbon monoxide poisoning)

e) Increased blood volume (sodium toxicity)

f) In rickets, interference with respiration

g) Secondary to liver damage

h) High altitude

Diagnosis

1) Can be prevented by reducing the bird's oxygen requirement.
2) Reducing feed, controlling environmental temperature and ventilation could be tried.
3) Controlling etiologic agents can prevent ascites caused by other factors (sodium, lung pathology, and liver damage).
4) Altitudes >1820m are unsatisfactory for broiler chickens.

72

Hypoglycemia-Spiking Mortality Syndrome of Broiler Chickens (HSMS)

Introduction

Hypoglycemia Spiking mortality syndrome is a disease in broilers, characterized by low mortality with sudden onset of high mortality. The affected birds are clinically hypoglycemic.

There is no known aetiology.

Clinical Signs

Clinical signs include ataxia, trembling, blindness, prostration and coma.

Gross Lesions

Gross lesions, although non-specific, are haemorrhages and necrosis in the liver. HSMS have depressed pancreatic glucagon levels. The chicks with HSMS show lower levels of glucagon and glycogen.

Diagnosis

Sudden mortality in 7-21 day old chicks is suggestive of HSMS. Typical clinical signs and hypoglycemia in the blood are (glucose lower than 150 mg/dL) reliable diagnostic feature.

Treatment, Prevention and Control

No treatment is known. Affected flocks are allowed to rest and fed a balanced diet. Controlled light and darkness program is helpful in the prevention of HSMS.

73

Proventricular Dilatation of Broiler Chickens

The condition is characterized by proventriculitis and dilatation of proventriculus.

Etiology

The cause of transmissible viral proventriculitis (TVP) is a birnavirus referred as Chicken proventricular necrosis virus (CPNV). TVP is a disease of 3-8 week-old broiler.

Clinical Signs

Clinical Signs include stunted growth and presence of undigested feed in faeces.

Lesions

Proventriculus is widened and thickened. Microscopically necrosis of glandular epithelial cells is a feature.

Diagnosis

1) Isolation and identification of CPNV.
2) FAT to detect antigen in the proventriculus.
3) RT-PCR is conducted for identification of CPNV.

Differential Diagnosis

Condition needs to be differentiated form agents causing proventriculitis and proventricular dilatation. These include copper sulphate ingestion, mycotoxins, reovirus, adenovirus, IBV, and bacteria.

74

Round Heart Disease of Chickens and Turkeys (Dilated cardiomyopathy)

Seen in mature chickens. Condition results from myocardial degeneration which causes bilateral ventricular hypertrophy and dilation. Etiology is not known.

Round heart disease in turkey causes mortality in 1-4 weeks of age. Lesions are severe cardiomyopathy, ascites, hydropericardium and generalized congestion of tissues. No aetiology is known.

Impacted or Egg bound oviducts

The condition is mostly observed in pullets that started early production before full body development. It is also seen in obese hens. Escherichia coli infection is also indicated as a cause of the condition. The oviduct is impacted with either one egg or mass of broken shells, or contents of many eggs (coagulated albumen, yolk, shell membranes). Impaction many times causes the presence of egg or egg material in the abdomen.

Clinical Signs

Clinical signs are not specific. However, hens are reluctant to move and have enlarged and pendulous abdomen.

Essential Conditions and Vices of birds

A. Territorial behavior

a) Fowls stay together as a group, in preferential areas of hen's house

b) Drive away others not belonging to their group

c) Domination

d) Weaker birds were driven away from feeder and waterer

e) Subordination

f) Weak layers become worthless

g) Weak cocks lose reproductive activity

h) Thus, feeding troughs, waterers and nests boxes

i) Should be distributed evenly in the poultry houses.

B. Feather Pecking

Chickens in some cases develop a habit (vice) of pulling feathers of others. Excessive pecking causes skin laceration, wound and mortality.

Etiology

a) Imbalanced diet (feed low in protein, minerals and vitamins)

b) Too intense light

c) Insufficient waterer and feeders in the poultry house

• Remedy

a) Apply repellent (1% iodine solution) on pecked areas

b) Debeaking:

    1) First in 7-10 days and second 9-12 weeks of age.

    2) Trim 1/3 of the beak length perpendicular to the long axis of separating the nostrils from the point of the beak.

C. Canabilism

Common forms of cannibalism are feather pulling, vent, head and toe picking. In over weight birds, normal eversion and prolapse of the vagina are usually occurs during lay. Cage mates attracted to the shiny red mucosa of vagina start mucosal picking. Toe picking is common in young chicks. Light intensity, heavy stocking density, lack of protein, minerals, vitamins, hunger, infestation with external parasites are predisposing factors. Once a bird develops a habit of cannibalism, it continues. For control of cannibalism regulate the light intensity and provide balanced feed.

D. Moulting (shedding of feathers)

It is natural physiological phenomenon.

• Consequences

a) Slowing down of laying or even complete halt of laying

b) Followed by renewed growth of feathers

c) also occurs accidentally

• Natural moulting

• 1st moult

a) Begins at 6-8 days; ends at four weeks

b) Down feathers are changed to 1st juvenile plumage

• 2nd moult

a) Occurs between 7 and 12 weeks; lasts for several weeks

b) 1st juvenile plumage changed to 2nd juvenile plumage

• 3rd moult

a) Real moult; "the moult."

b) Occurs during 16 to 18 months of age : affects neck , head , breast , tail and wings

c) Hen stops laying

d) Accidental moulting

• Results when there is:

a) Defective ventilation

b) Overcrowding

c) Shortage of water or feed

d) Excessive heat

• Effects of moulting

Economic loss to the farmer

• Induced moulting

By holding feed for 4-6 days and reducing light, usually done at the end of first laying cycle (72 weeks of age).

To lessen the duration of moult use following.

a) Feeding layers with a perfectly balanced ration.

b) Administration of iodothyroxine (60g/100 kg feed) for 3-4 weeks.

After this moult, layers start laying again at a satisfactory level.

Colour Plates

Chapter 4: Avian Salmonellosis

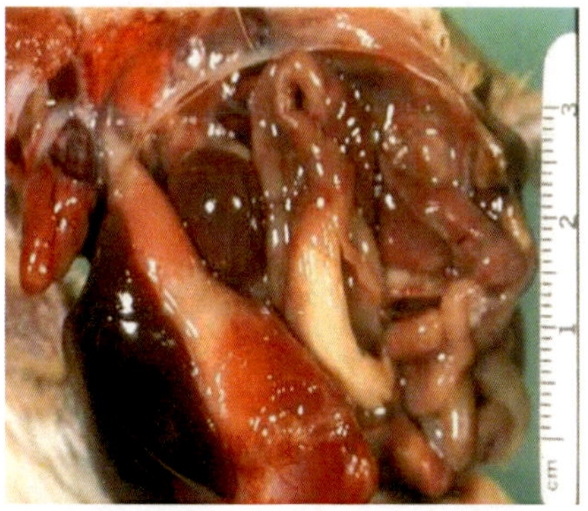

Fig. 1: *S. Pullorum/gallinarum* in 18 day-old chick (liver and spleen enlarged and congested, white cast in the cecum)

Fig. 2: *S. Pullorum/gallinarum* (hock joint synovitis)

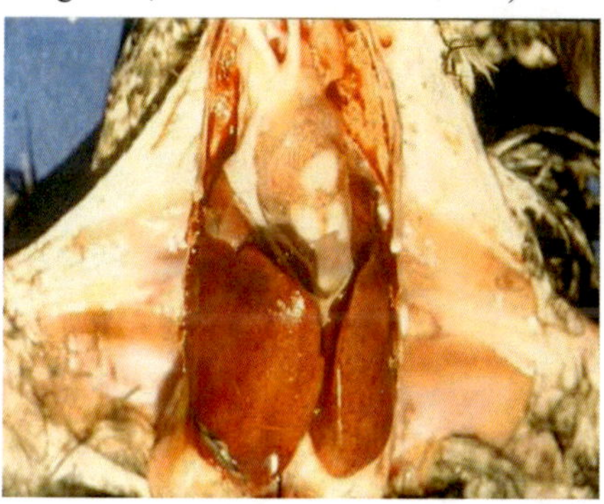

Fig. 3: *S. Pullorum/gallinarum*; 5 wk-old-chick (3 white nodules resembling tumors in the heart. Liver enlarged and congested).

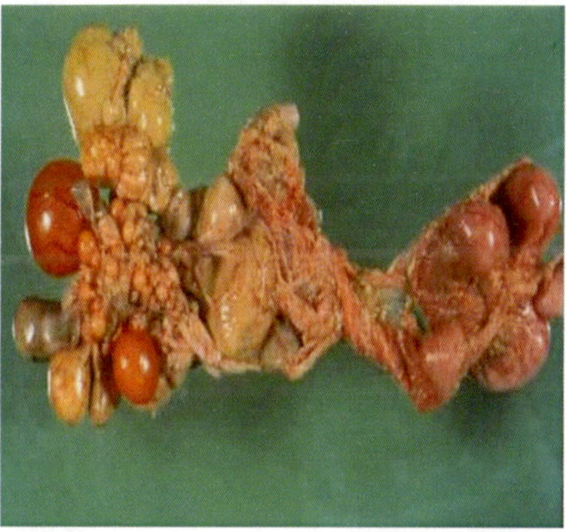

Fig . 4: *S. Pullorum/gallinarum;* Adult chicken (ovary with many misshapen nodular gray to yellow follicles)

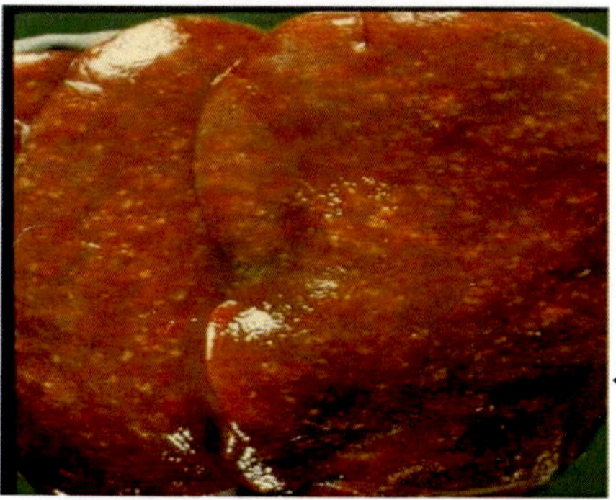

← **Fig. 5:** *S. Pullorun/gallinarum* in adult chicken (enlarged liver with multifocal necrosis)

Chapter 7: Avian Mycoplasmosis

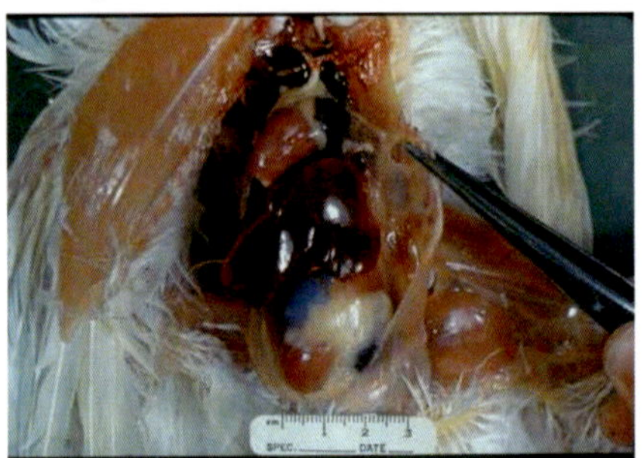

Fig.7: Chicken. Air saculitis seen as thickened air sac membrane.

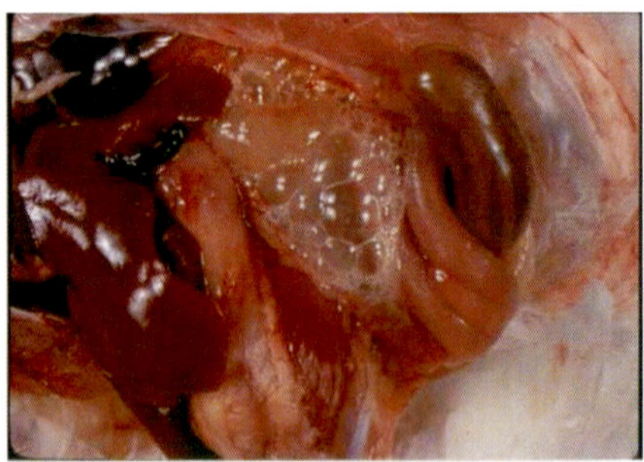

Fig. 8: Chicken. Lesions of air saculitis in abdominal air sac

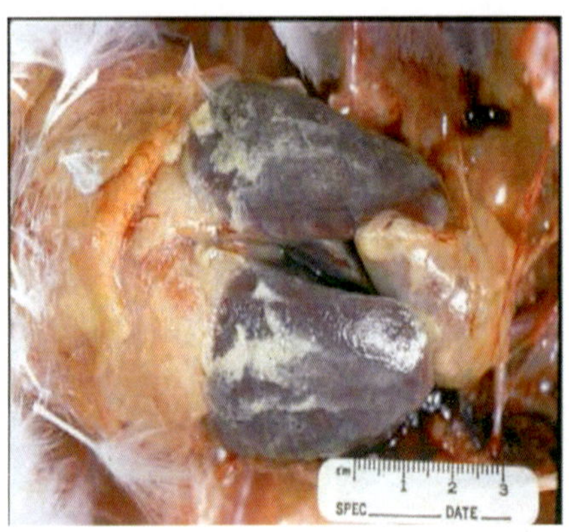

Fig. 9: Complicated *Mycoplasma gallisepticum* infection (pericarditis and perihepatitis)

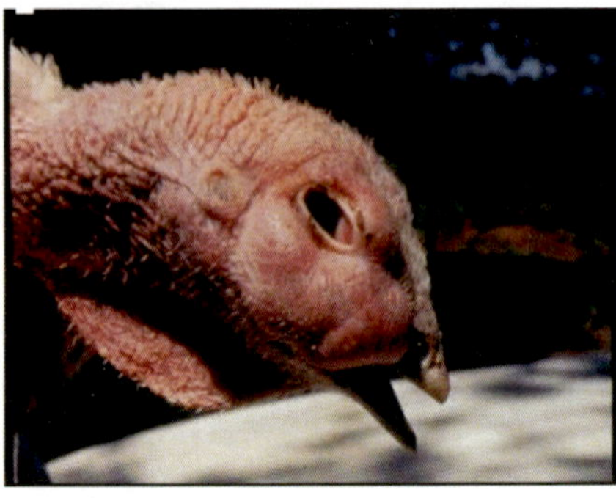

Fig. 10: *Mycoplasma gallisepticum* in turkey (swollen sinuses- infectious sinusitis)

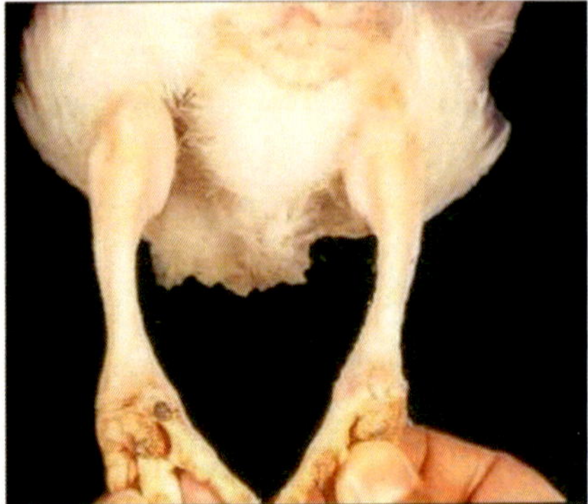

Fig. 11: *M. meleagridis*; 3-wk-old turkey poult with bowing of tarso-metatarsal bone.

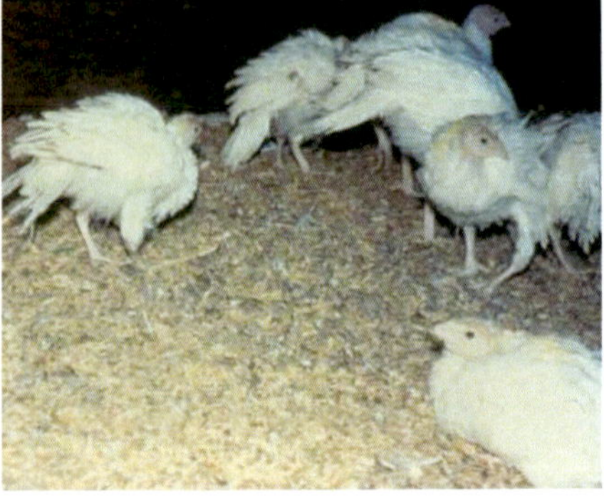

Fig.12: 10-wks-old turkey poults with swelling of hock joint infected with *M. meleagridis*.

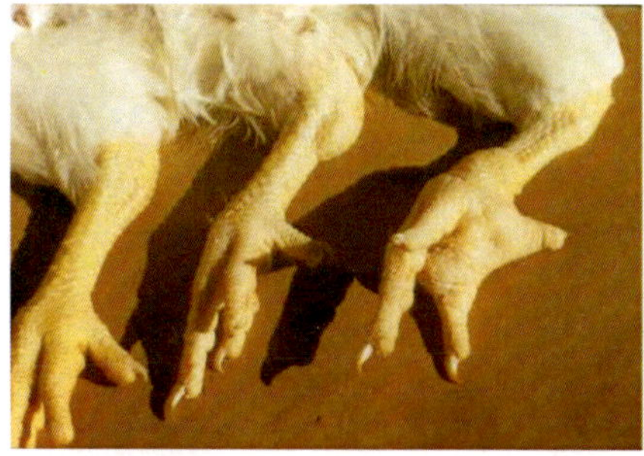

Fig. 13: *Mycoplasma synoviae* infection typical lesion- swollen foot pads.

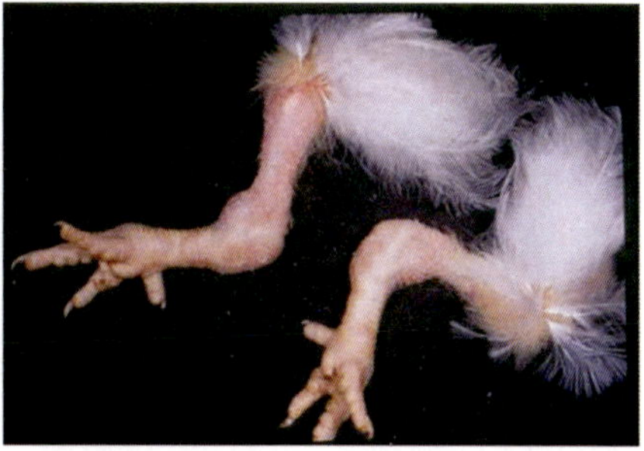

Fig. 14: Swollen hock and foot pads in MS infection.

Chapter 8: Colibacillosis / *Escherichia Coli* Infections

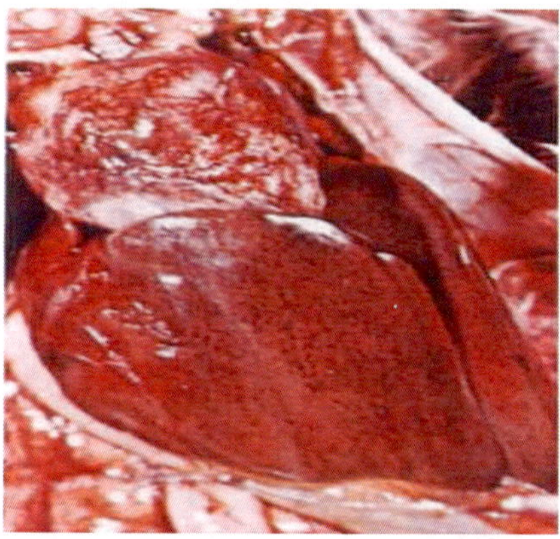

Fig. 15: *E. Coli* infection- enlarged mottled liver and pericarditis.

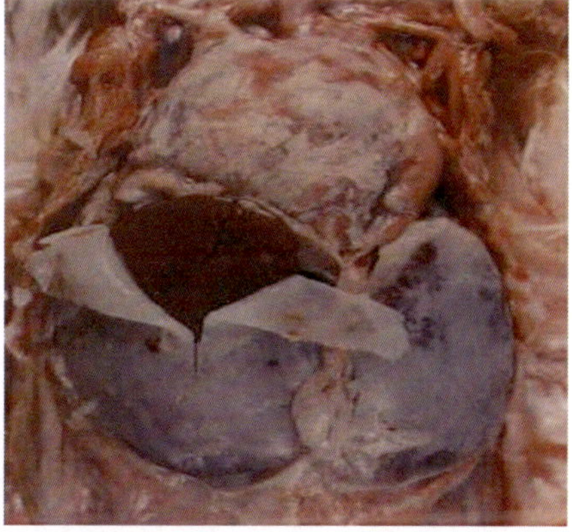

Fig. 16: *E. coli*/mycoplasma complicated case. Severe pericarditis and perihepatitis.

Chapter 9: Fowl Cholera

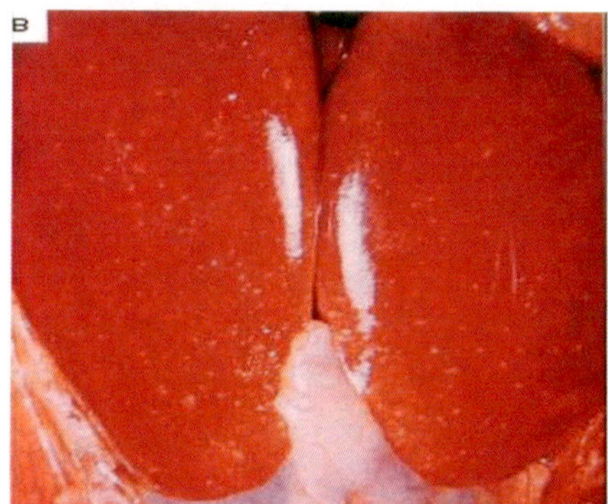

Fig. 17: Liver from a turkey showing enlargement, congestion and multiple white necrotic foci in acute fowl cholera.

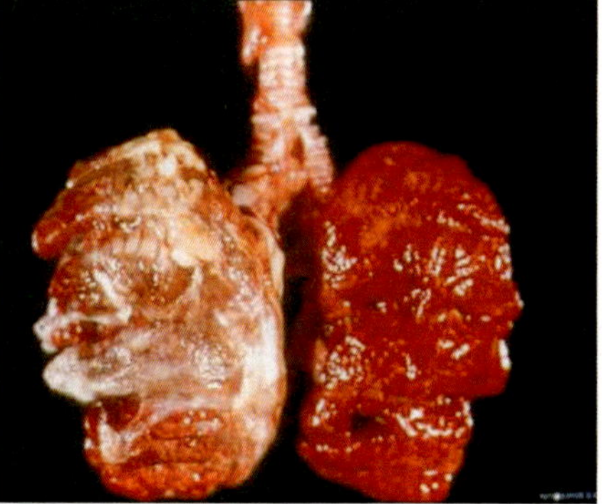

Fig. 18: Unilateral fibrinous pleuritis and pneumonia in turkey in acute fowl cholera.

Chapter 16: Clostridial Infections

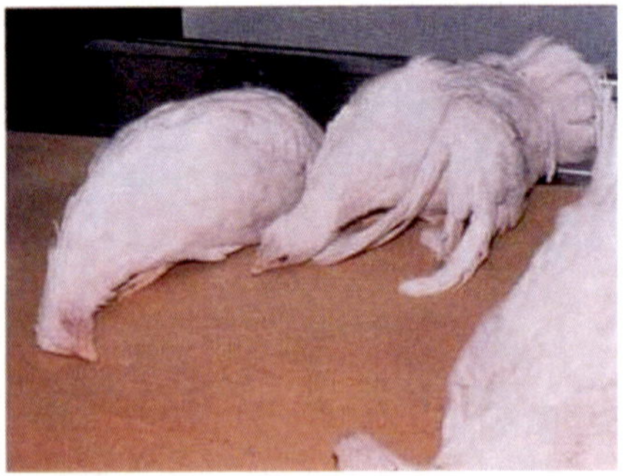

Fig.19: *Clostridium botulinum* infection. Birds showing "limberneck" characteristic of Botulism.

Chapter 17: Infectious Coryza (Fowl Coryza)

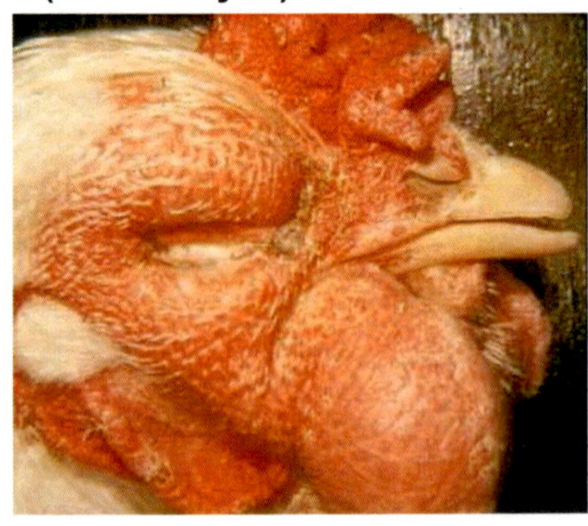

Fig. 20: Infectious coryza; edema of face, wattles and around the eyes causing closing of the eye

Chapter 20: Mycobacteriosis

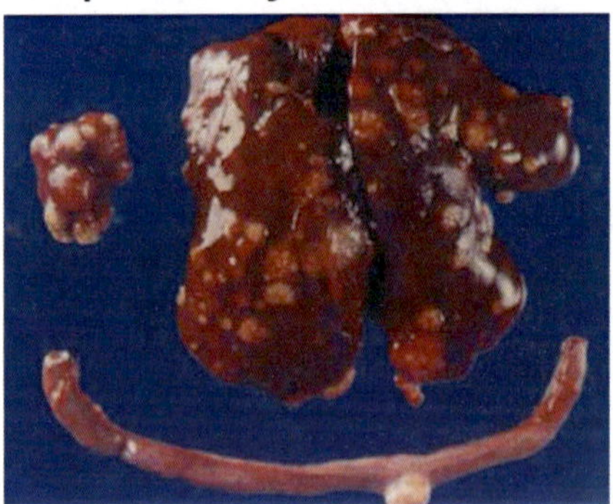

Fig. 21: Mycobacteriosis (yellowish caseous nodules in liver, intestine and spleen)

Chapter 21: Chlamydiosis

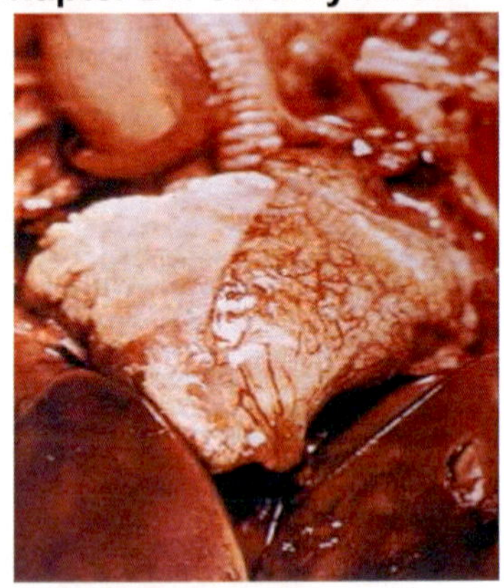

Fig. 22: Chlamydiosis in a turkey (pericarditis, enlarged liver)

Fig. 23: Chlamydia species stained with Giemsa; organisms seen in mononuclear cells. →

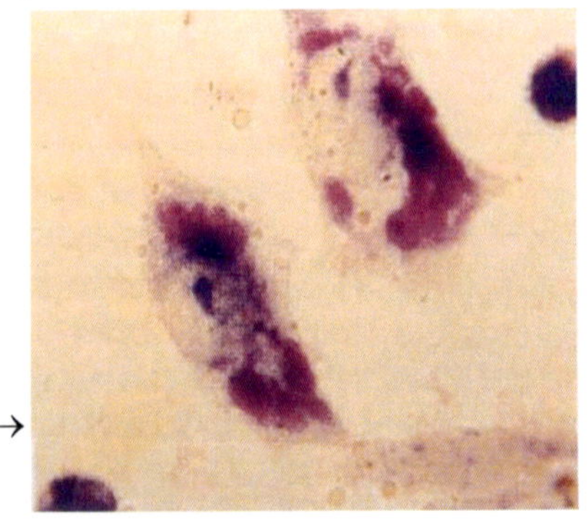

Chapter 22: Omphalitis (Navel ill, Mushy chick disease)

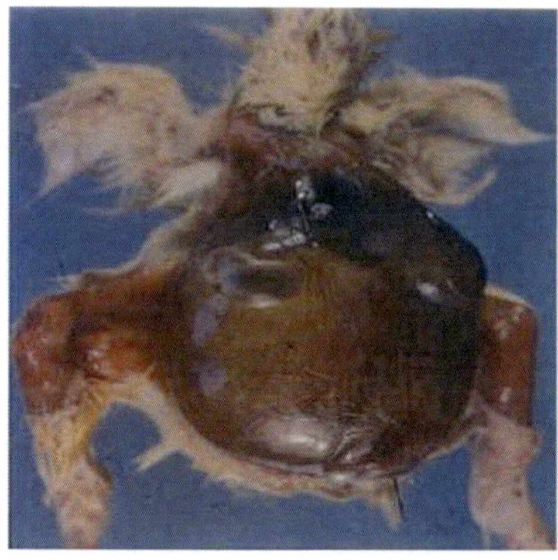

Fig. 24: Omphalitis (abdomen is greatly distended as a result of yolk sac infection)

Chapter 26: Newcastle Disease (ND; Avian Pneumoencephalitis)

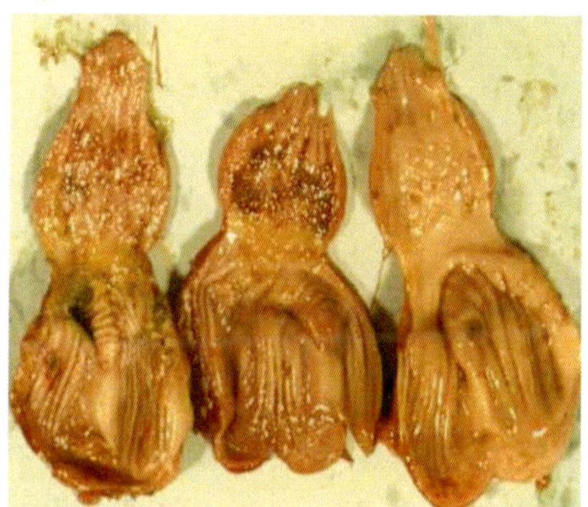

Fig. 25: Newcastle disease; Hemorrhages in the proventriculus

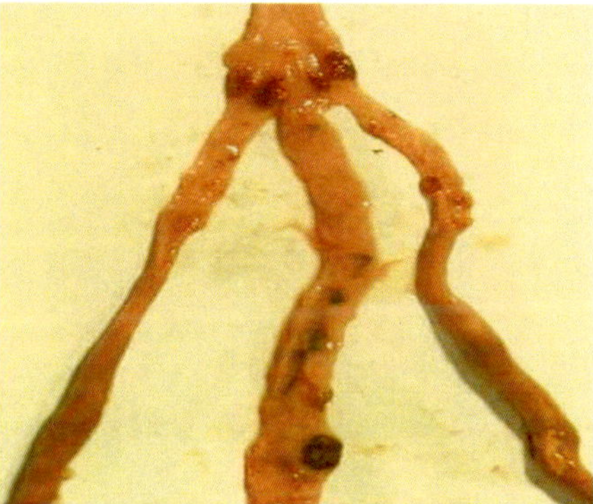

Fig. 26: Newcastle disease; Hemorrhages in the cecal tonsils and intestinal mucosa

Chapter 28: Infectious Laryngotracheitis (Laryngotracheitis, ILT; LT)

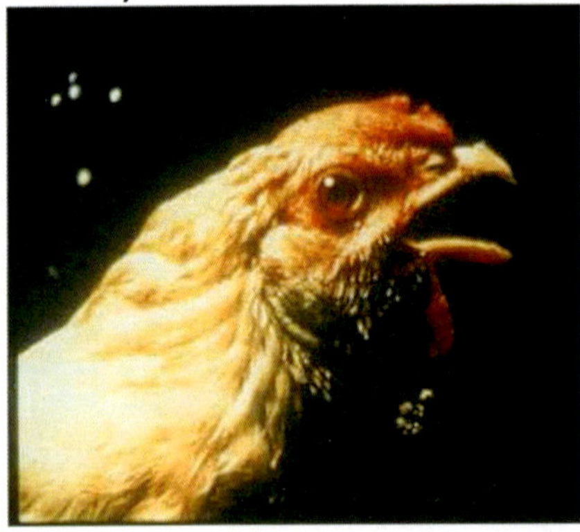

Fig. 27: ILT; Chicken showing difficult breathing.

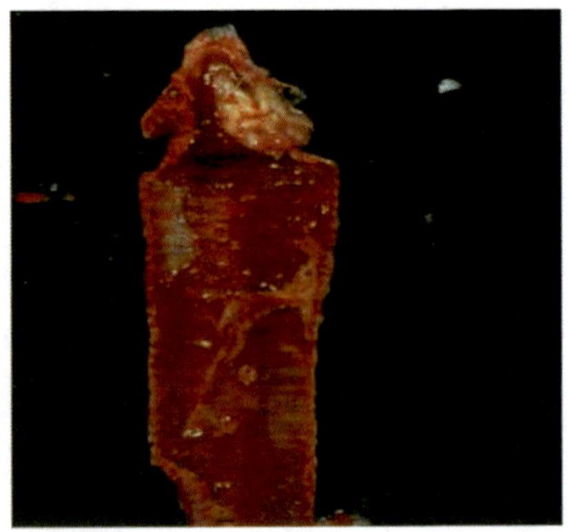

Fig. 28: ILT; Acute form, hemorrhagic trachea.

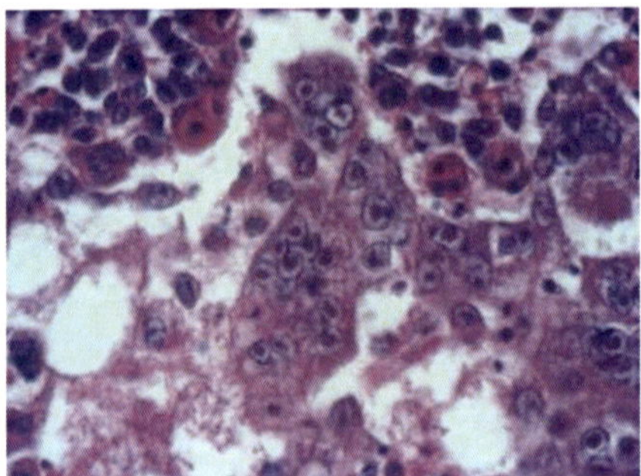

Fig. 29: ILT; Intra-nuclear inclusions seen in the sloughed epithelial cells of the trachea

Chapter 29: Infectious Bronchitis (IB)

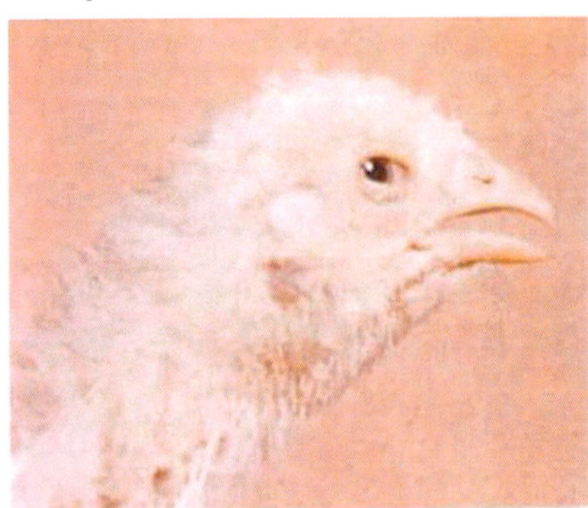

Fig. 30: IB; Chick breathing through mouth as a result of swollen sinuses,

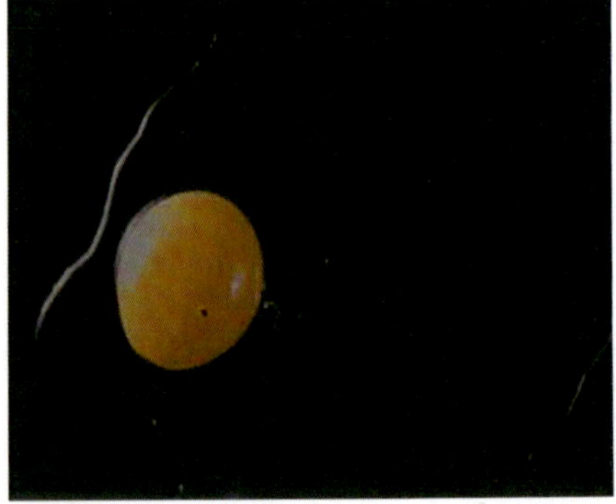

Fig. 31: IB; Changes in the internal quality of egg; albumen becomes watery.

Chapter 30: Infectious Anemia (Chicken Anemia Agent [CAA] infection)

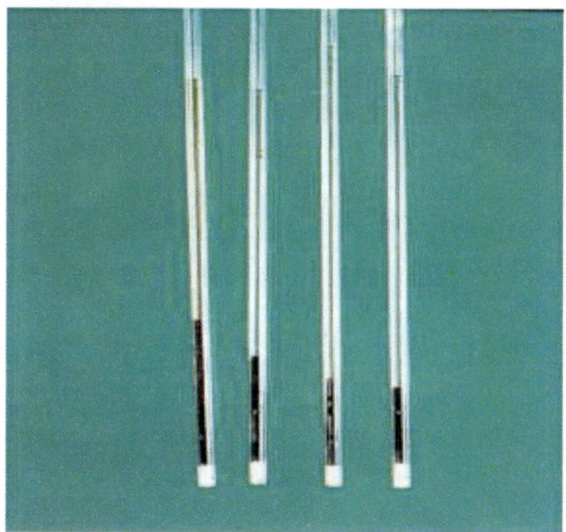

Fig. 32: Chicken infectious anemia virus infection; low hematocrit value in infected chicken

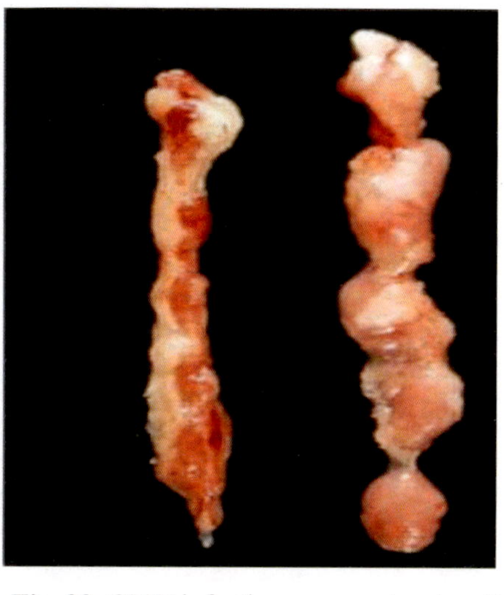

Fig. 33: CIAV infection; severe atrophy of thymus compared to normal thymus at the right,

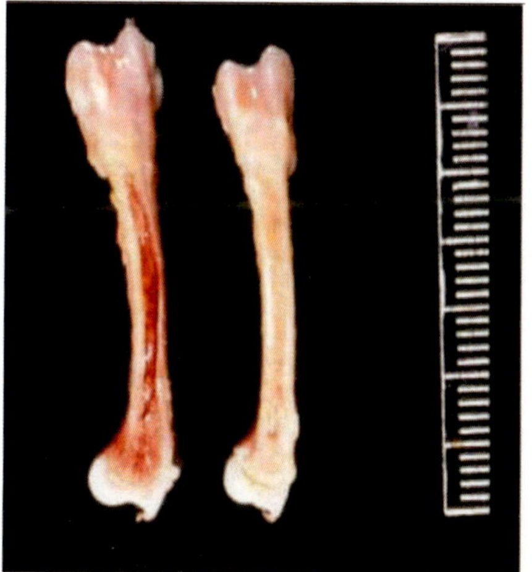

Fig. 34: CIAV infection; pale yellow fatty marrow (right) compared to normal marrow

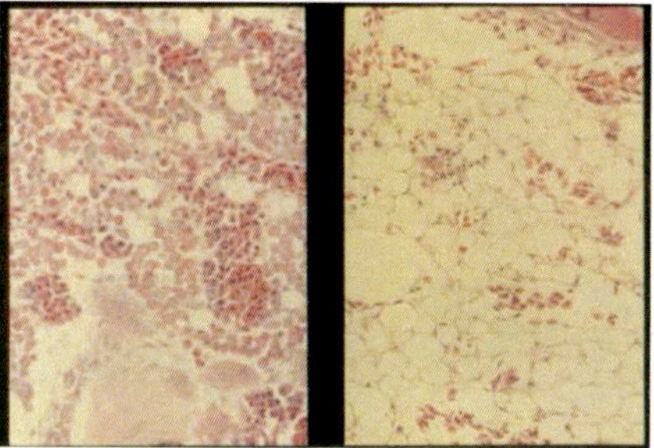

Fig. 35: CIAV infection; severe hypoplasia of erythroid and myeloid cells and replacement by adipose tissue, compared to normal on the left.

Chapter 36: Viral Arthritis

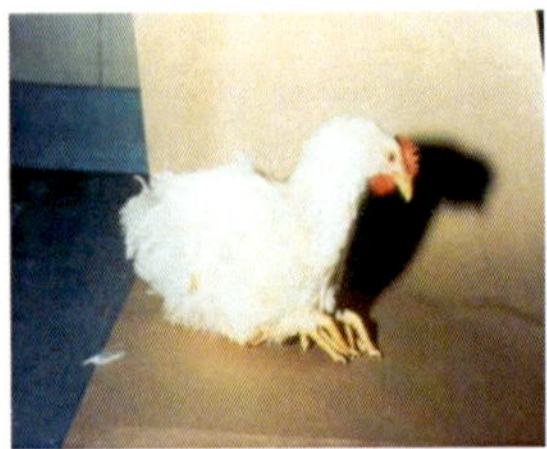

Fig. 37: Viral arthritis; Chicken with tendo-sinovitis, prefers to sit and reluctant to move

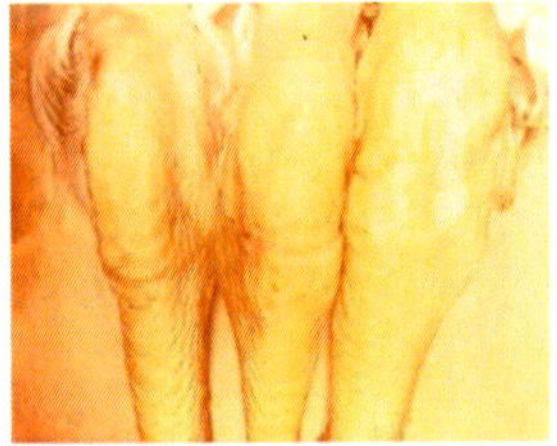

Fig. 38: Viral arthritis; Swelling of tendon sheath above the hock joint- a characteristic lesion;

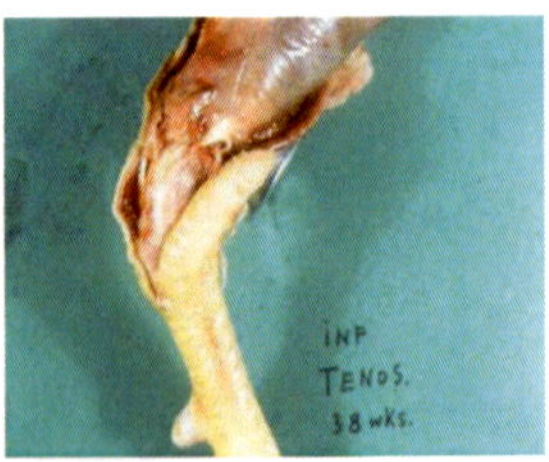

Fig. 39: Viral arthritis; Rupture of gastrocnemius tendon

Chapter 37: Fowl Pox (Pox; Avian Pox)

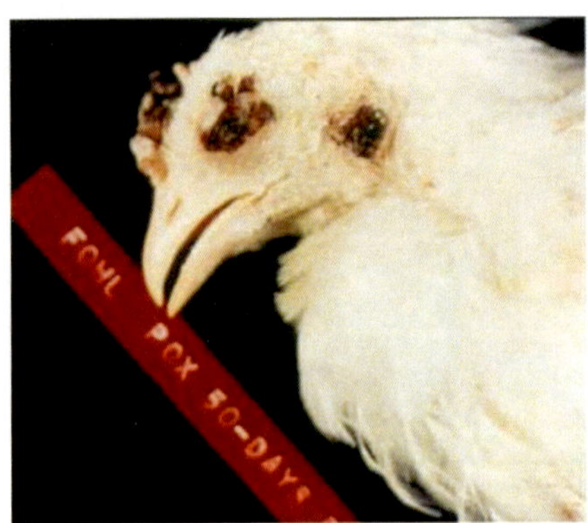

Fig.40: Fowl pox; Cutaneous lesions on comb and eye lids;

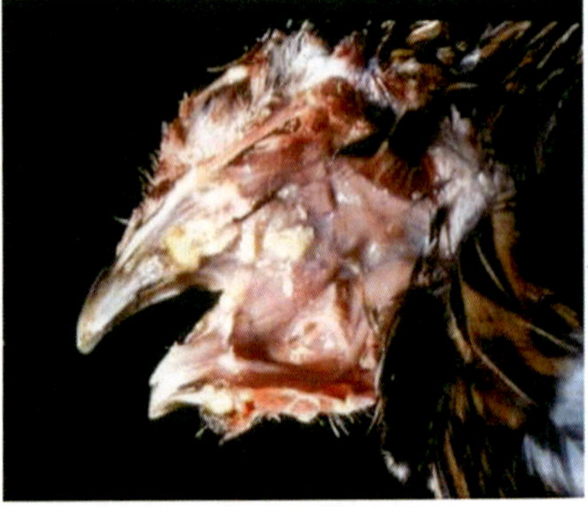

Fig. 41: Fowl pox; Diphtheritic lesions in the mouth cavity

Chapter 38: Infectious Bursal Disease (IBD; Gumboro Disease)

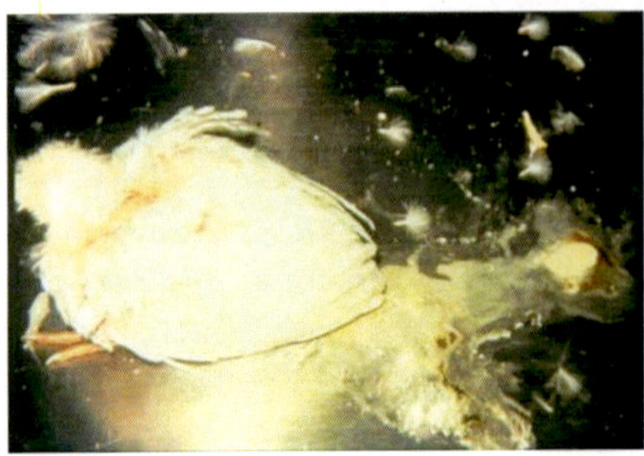

Fig. 42: IBD; Infected chicken is typically depressed showing ruffled feathers and watery diarrhea

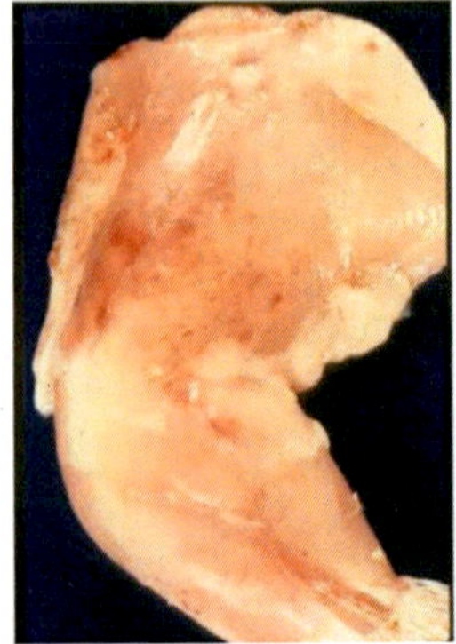

Fig. 43: IBD; Hemorrhages into the thigh muscles

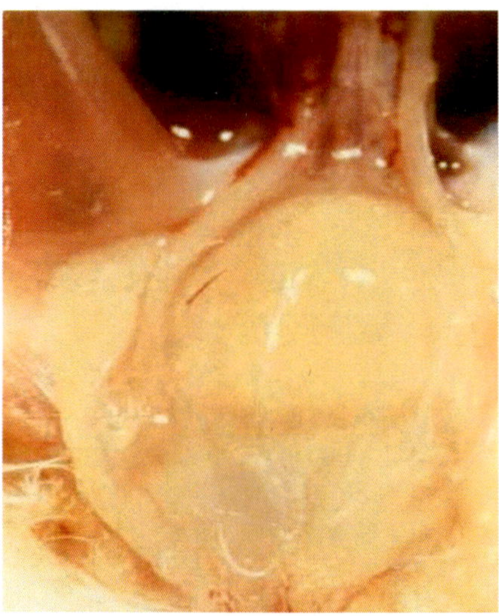

Fig. 44: IBD; Swollen and edematous bursa, 2-3 day PI

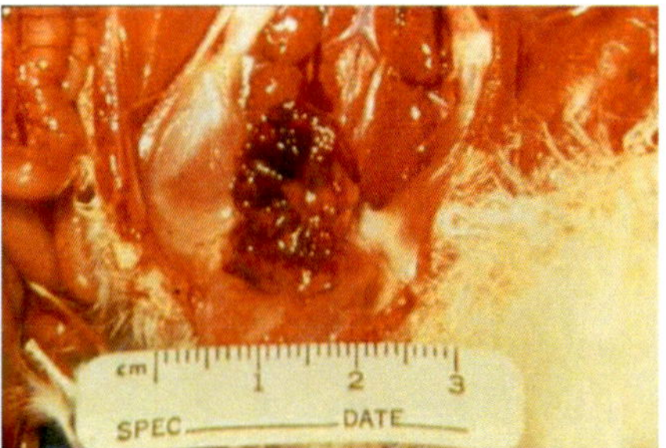

Fig. 45: IBD; In some outbreaks bursa exhibits extensive hemorrhages in the lumen

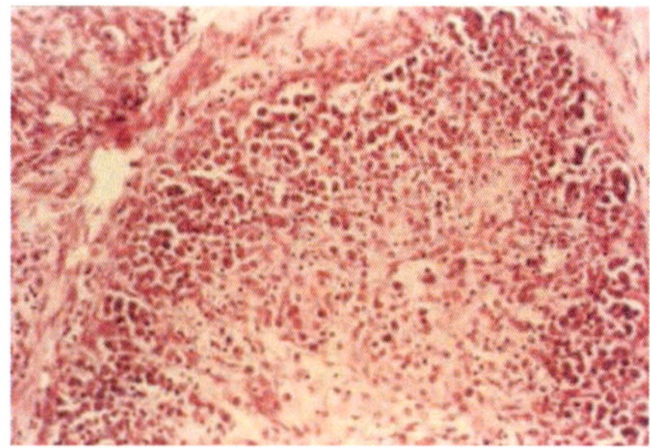

Fig. 46: IBD; Necrosis of the bursal follicles

Chapter 39: Marek's Disease

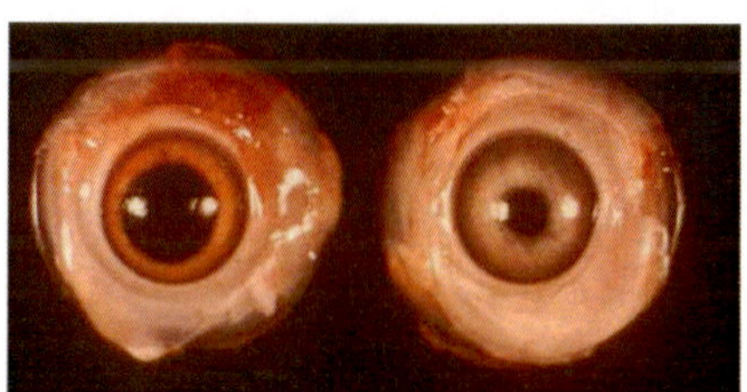

Fig. 47: MD. Eye lesions-Cellular infiltration in iris (right) causing white discoloration. Pupil is irregular and does not respond to light intensity

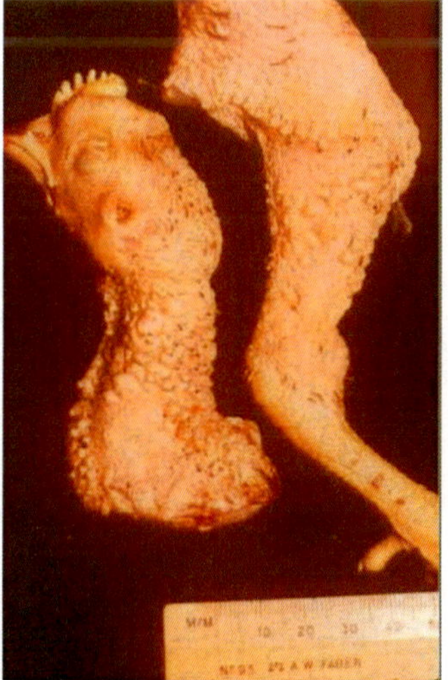

Fig. 49: MD. Tumors marked on the skin,

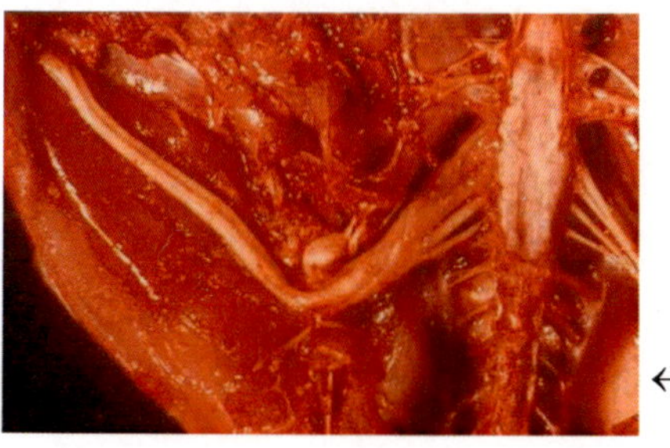

← **Fig. 48:** MD. Involved sciatic nerve is thickened, dull and yellowish in contrast to glistening white unaffected right nerve

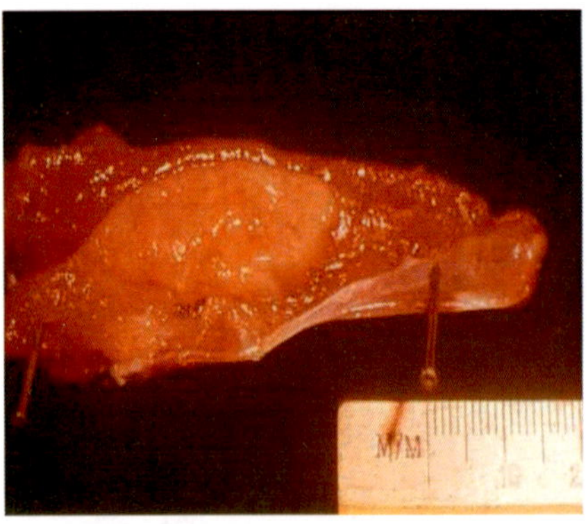

Fig. 50: MD. Tumor in the muscle

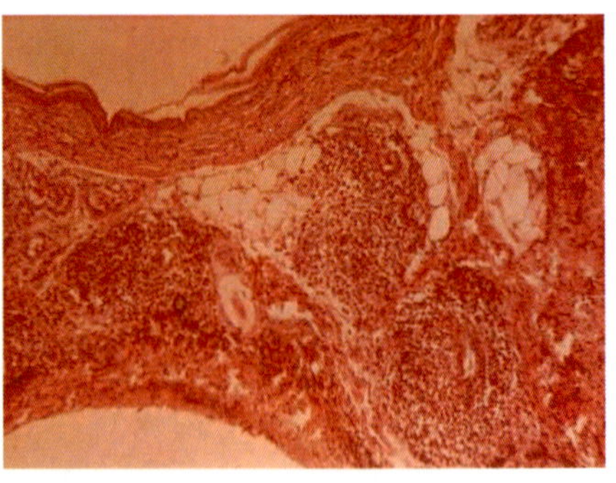

Fig. 51: MD. Microscopic lesions in the skin, infiltration of pleomorphic lymphoid cells around the hair follicles and below the epidermis,

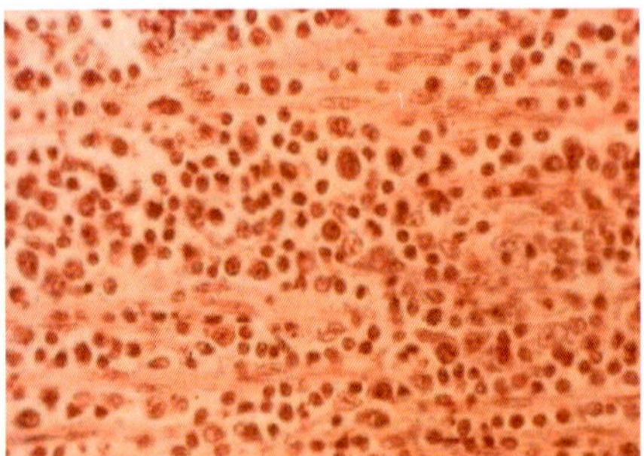

Fig. 52: MD. Microscopic lesions-pleomorphic lymphoid cells infiltration

Chapter 48: Duck Virus Enteritis (DVE, Duck Plague)

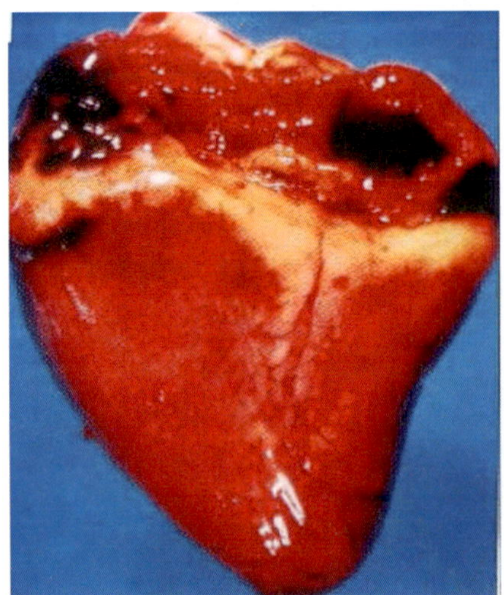

Fig. 56: DVE lesions; petechial hemorrhages on the epicardium

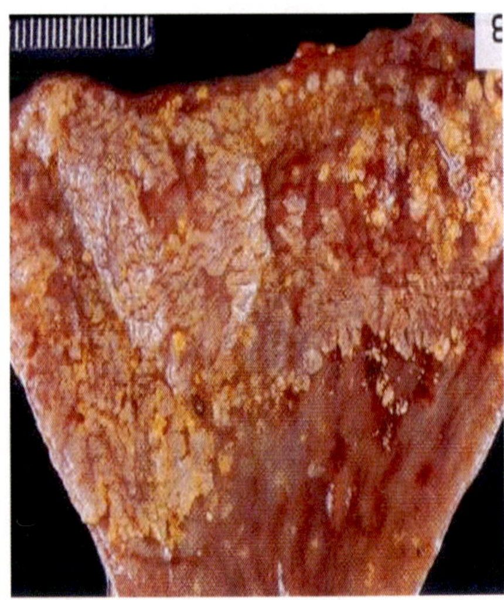

Fig. 57: DVE; extensive ulceration of esophageal mucosa

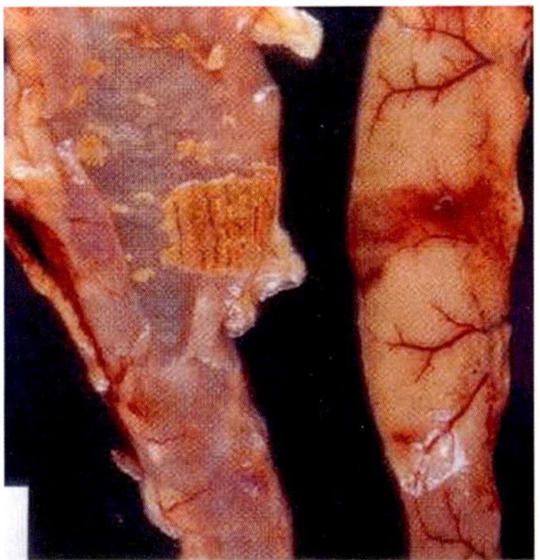

Fig. 58: DVE; band of red hemorrhagic areas on the serosal surface of the intestine, necrosis of GALT and ulceration,

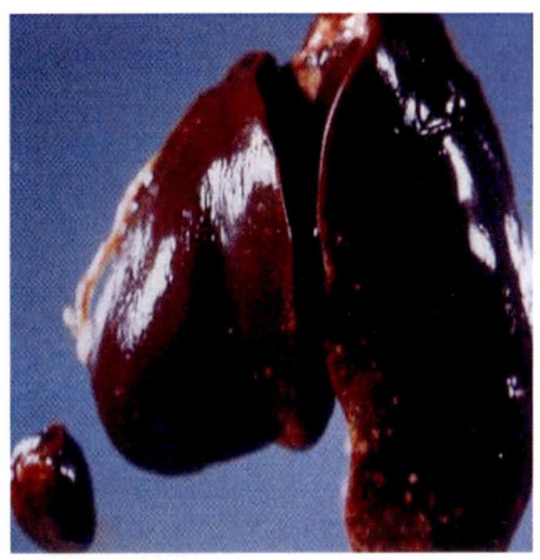

Fig. 59: DVE; multiple necrotic foci in the liver

Chapter 49: Duck Virus Hepatitis (DVH)

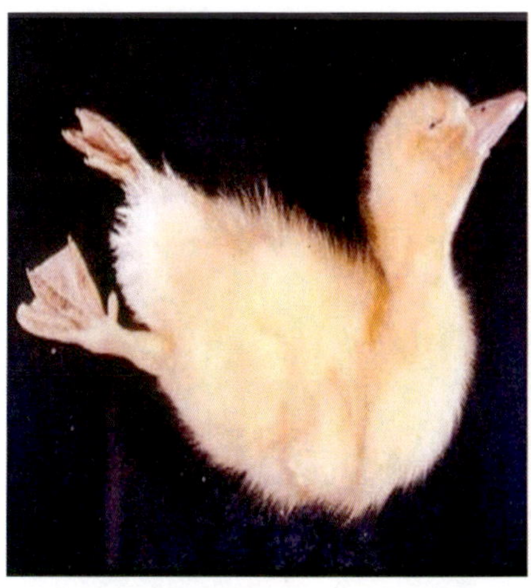

Fig. 60: Duck virus hepatitis (DVH); typical opisthotonos

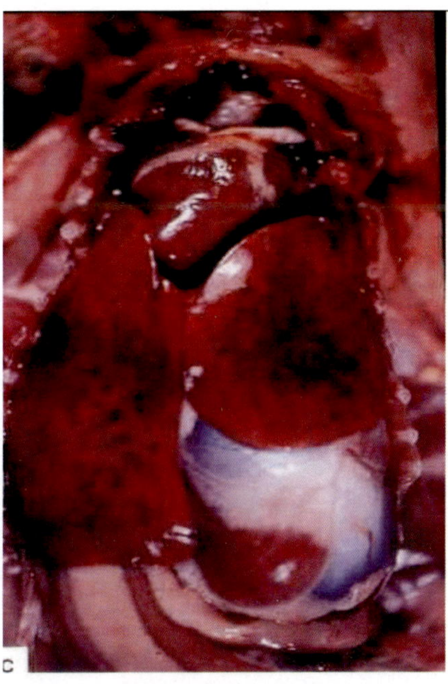

Fig. 61: DVH; massive hemorrhage and mottling of the liver

Chapter 52: Aspergillosis (Brooder pneumonia)

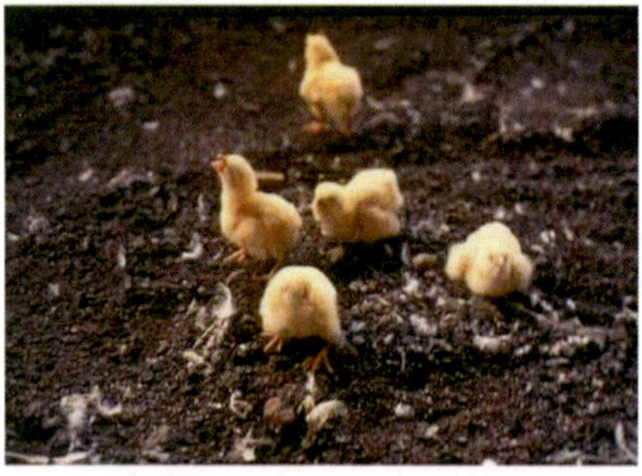

Fig. 62: Aspergillosis. Typical clinical signs (gasping)

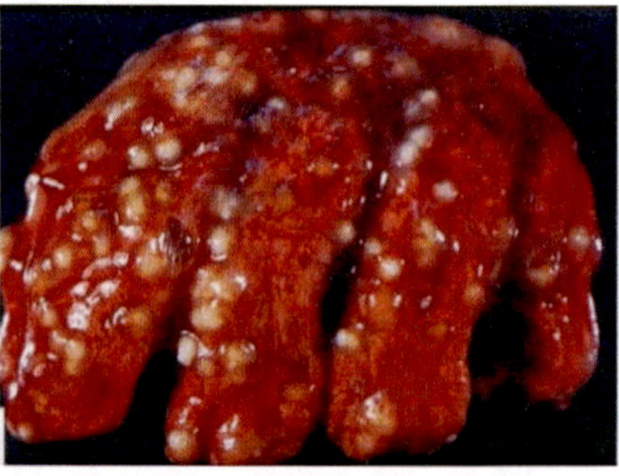

Fig. 63: Aspergillosis. White nodular lesions in the lung,

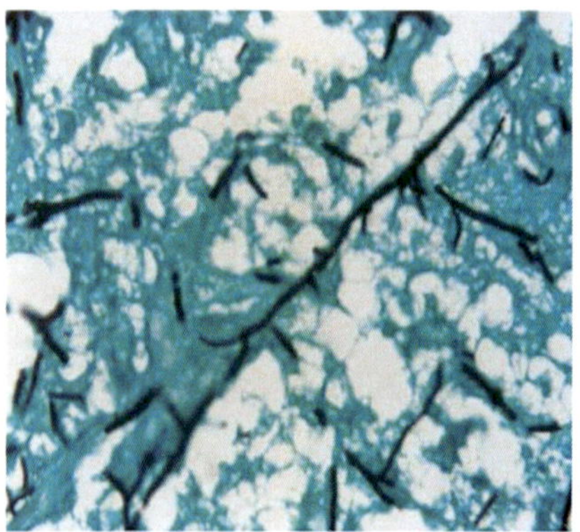

← **Fig. 64:** Aspergillosis. Mycelia of fungus in the lesion

Chapter 57: Coccidiosis

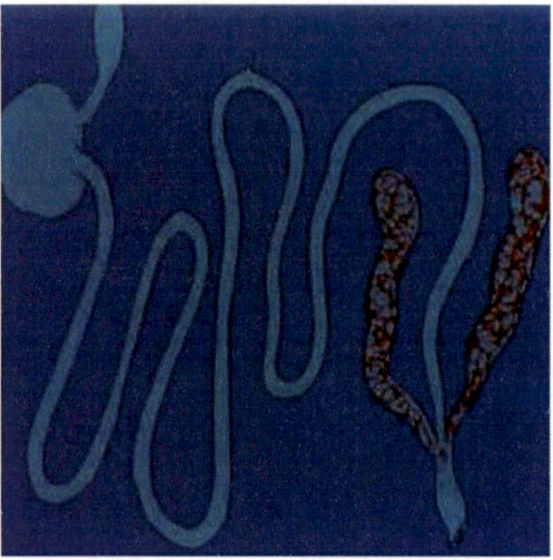

Fig. 66: Location of *E. tenella* infection; confined to ceca,

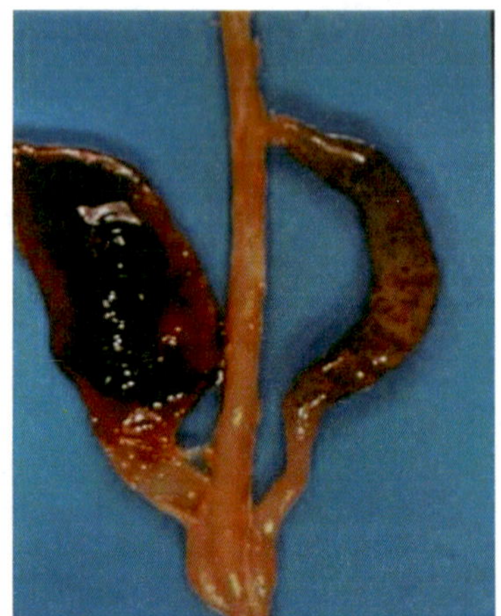

Fig. 67: *E. Tenella* infection; ceca distended with blood, petechial hemorrhages on serosa.

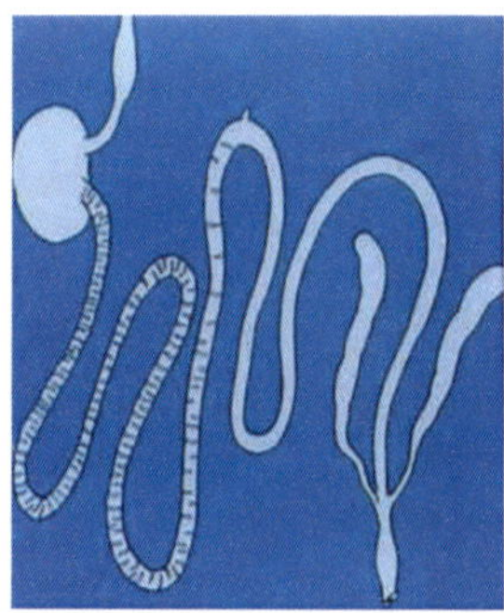

Fig. 68: Coccidiosis. Location of *E. acervulina* infections in the chicken-upper intestinal tract,

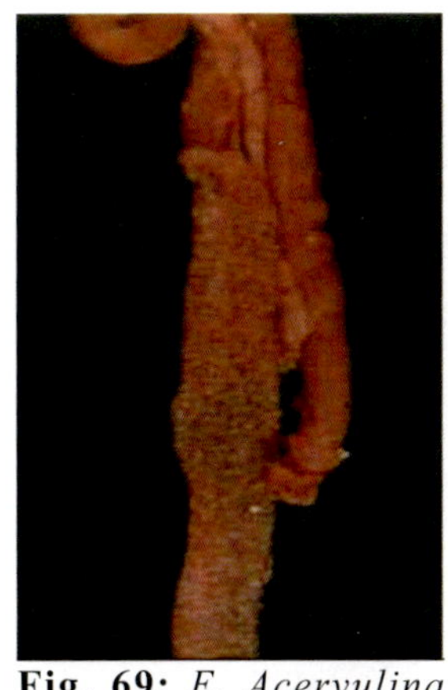

Fig. 69: *E. Acervulina* infection. Lesions are in the form of transverse bands, giving intestine a coated appearance

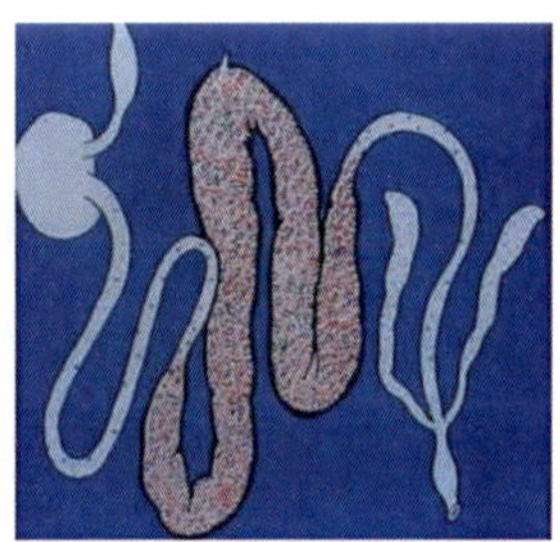

Fig. 70: Location of *E. necatrix* infection, usually mid intestine,

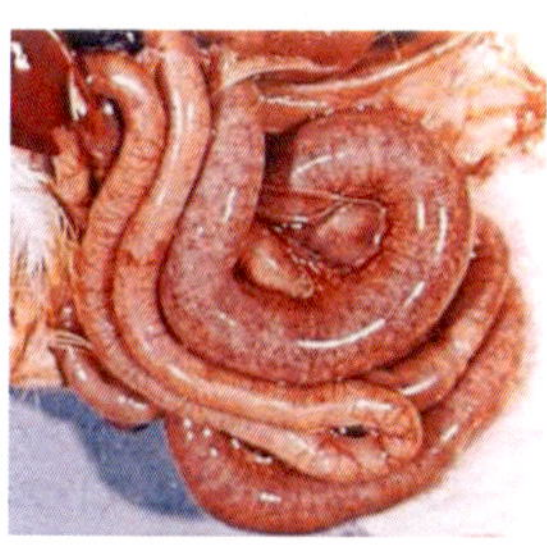

Fig. 71: *E. Necatrix* infection. Lesions consist of extremely ballooning and hemorrhage areas are clearly seen without opening the intestine; classic "salt and pepper" lesions on the serosal surface.

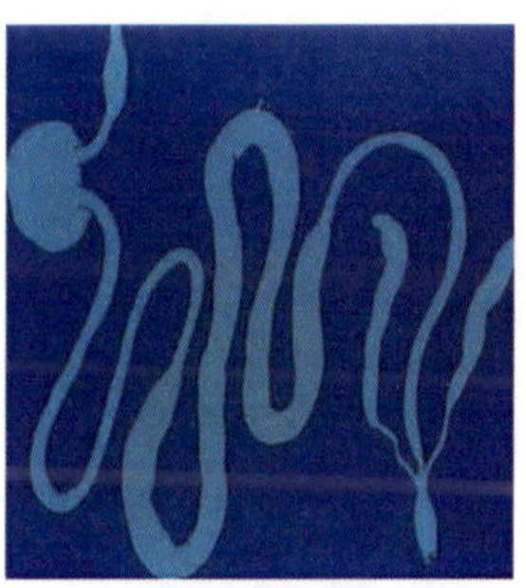

Fig. 72: Location of *E. maxima* infection, usually in the middle of the intestine but may extend to either side,

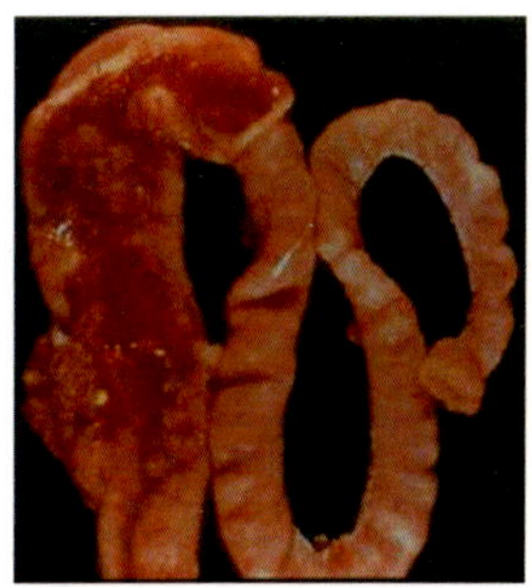

Fig. 73: *E. Maxima* infection. Lesions as red descrete hemorrhage on the serosal surface and orange mucus in the lumen.

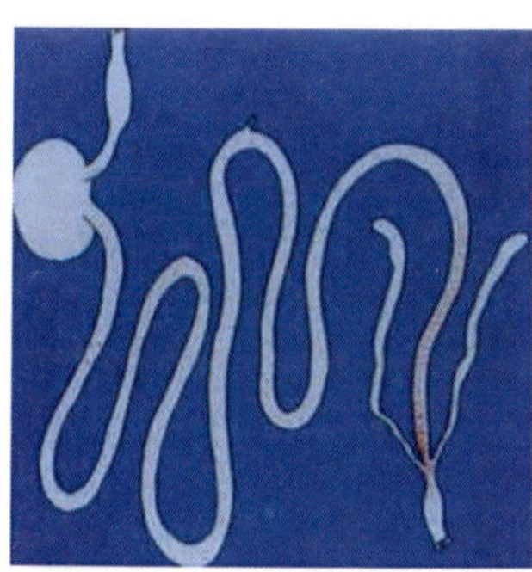

← **Fig. 74:** Location of *E. brunetti* infection; lower small intestine

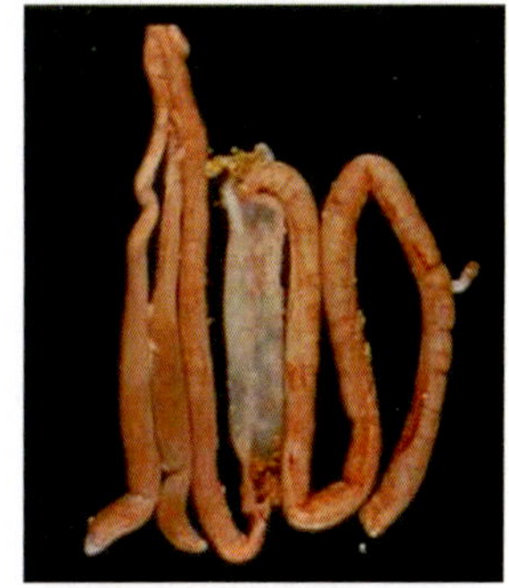

Fig. 75: *E. Brunetti* infection; lumen of lower small intestine contains hemorrhagic and mucoid content, ulcers seen in severe cases

Chapter 66: Vitamin Deficiency

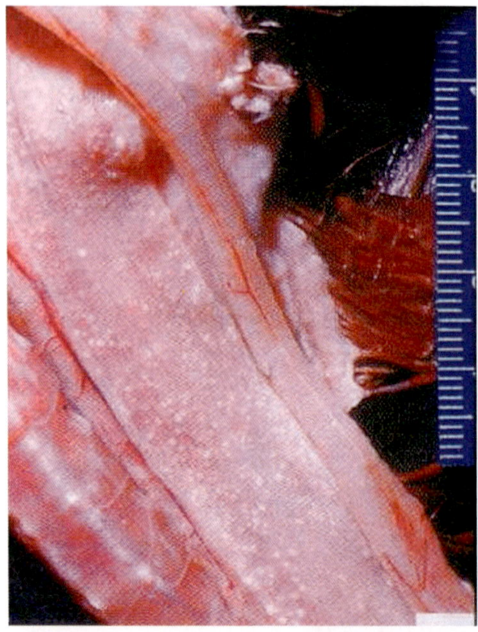

Fig. 76: Vitamin A deficiency; distended impacted mucosal glands resembling pustules in the esophagus.

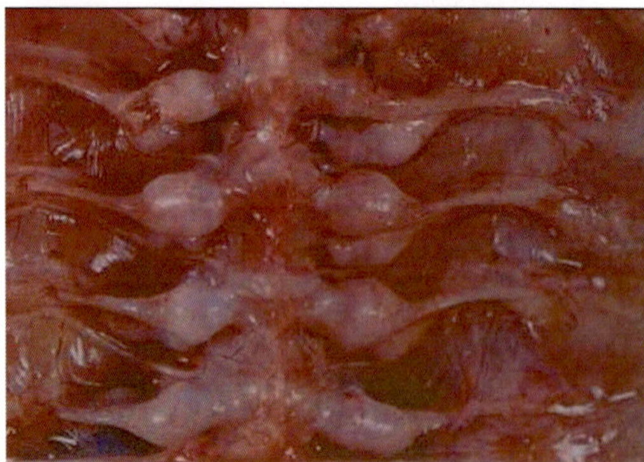

Fig. 77: Vitamin D deficiency; lesions of rickets rosary (beading of rib head),

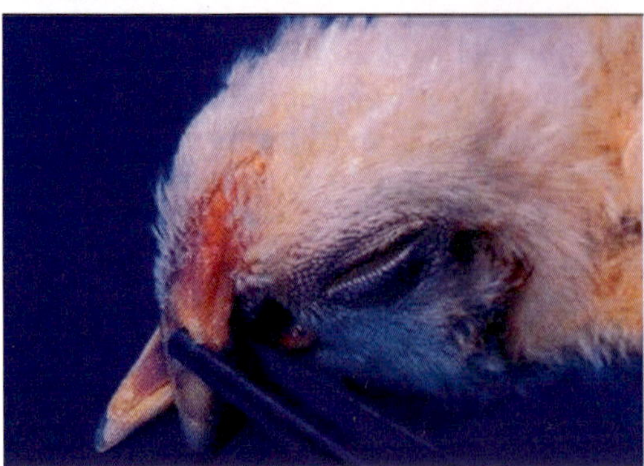

Fig. 78: Vitamin D deficiency; softening and bending of the beak

Index

I

L

M

N

O

P

Q

R

S

T

U

V,W,Y